PRAISE FOR

ISA CHANDRA MOSKOWITZ & TERRY HOPE ROMERO

VEGAN COOKIES INVADE YOUR COOKIE JAR

"[The] ultimate cookie manual." —*VegNews*

⁂

"Winning ... decadent recipes ... show that you can be vegan and still indulge in delicious treats." —*Publishers Weekly*

⁂

"Moskowitz and Romero are icons in the vegan world ... All your favorite cookies are here, alongside many that are about to become your favorites." —*Bar Harbor Times*

⁂

"An outstanding, surprisingly simple cookbook." —*Midwest Book Review*

⁂

"Will satisfy almost everyone's sweet tooth and visions of sugarplums."
—*Auburn Citizen*

VEGAN CUPCAKES TAKE OVER THE WORLD

"[Moskowitz and Romero] produce insanely fetching cupcakes with mousse fillings, butter cream frostings, chocolate ganache icings and sprinkles galore."
—*New York Times*

"Packed with 75 dairy-free recipes and lush photos aimed at making vegans and omnivores drool." —*Washington Post*

❧

"Written chattily and supportively for even the most oven-phobic ... reading this is like having a couple of fun, socially conscious post-punk pals over for a slumber party ... Each page of this cookbook contains an irresistible delight."
—*Bust*

VEGANOMICON

"The very same urban chefs who had you inhaling vegan butter-cream frosting during your free time have crafted the next revolution in neo-vegan cuisine."
—*Philadelphia City Paper*

❧

"Exuberant and unapologetic... recipes don't skimp on fat or flavor, and the eclectic collection of dishes is a testament to the authors' sincere love of cooking and culinary exploration."
—*Saveur*

❧

"The *Betty Crocker's Cookbook* of the vegan world." —*Bitch*

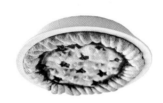

VEGAN PIE
IN THE SKY

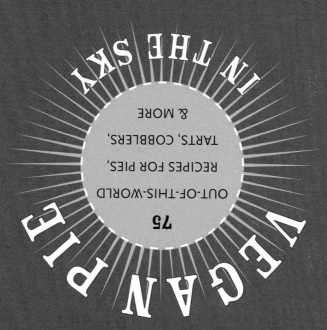

VEGAN PIE IN THE SKY

75
OUT-OF-THIS-WORLD
RECIPES FOR PIES,
TARTS, COBBLERS,
& MORE

ISA CHANDRA MOSKOWITZ & TERRY HOPE ROMERO

Da Capo
∞
LIFE
LONG

A MEMBER OF THE PERSEUS BOOKS GROUP

Copyright © 2011 by Isa Chandra Moskowitz and Terry Hope Romero

Text and photography copyright © 2011 by Isa Chandra Moskowitz and Terry Hope Romero

Editorial production by Marathon Production Services, www.marrathon.net
Adapted from original design by Pauline Neuwirth & Associates, Inc.
Set in 10.5 point Whitman

Cataloging-in-Publication Data for this book is available from the Library of Congress.

ISBN 978-0-7382-1274-6 (paperback)
ISBN 978-0-7382-1535-8 (e-Book)

Published by Da Capo Press
A Member of the Perseus Books Group
www.dacapopress.com

Da Capo Press books are available at special discounts for bulk
purchases in the U.S. by corporations, institutions, and other organizations.
For more information, please contact the Special Markets Department at the Perseus
Books Group, 2300 Chestnut Street, Suite 200, Philadelphia, PA, 19103, or call
(800) 810-4145, ext. 5000, or e-mail special.markets@perseusbooks.com.

First Da Capo Press edition 2011

10 9 8 7 6 5 4 3 2

In memory of
ADRIENNE SHELLEY,
who celebrated life, love, and pie

CONTENTS

INTRODUCTION

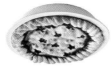

THERE ARE FEW MOMENTS in life that can't be improved with a slice of pie. Cakes and cookies and even cupcakes are iconic in their own right, but pie says "sit down, feel right at home, you're with friends now." Not just layers of pastry and filling, pie is comforting and approachable, yet entirely enticing. Can you picture Agent Cooper from *Twin Peaks* waxing over a piece of angel food cake? No way. His black coffee must come saddled with a slice of honest cherry pie.

Pie is the perfect fusion of art, craft, and kitchen, unlike anything else you can bake in your oven today. Or right now. That's correct; we feel that anyone should be able to bake a pie whenever the situation calls for it, no matter what their level of experience. Requiring little in the way of equipment, but a worth-while investment of time, pies can easily become a way of life.

The kind of person that just *makes* pie, simply because that's what they *do*, is a station apart from the hurried, stressed-out masses reaching for instant sugar rushes and quick fixes. Learn how to make a pie and really take your time to enjoy doing it; it's as calming as a yoga class or a day at the beach.

Pie, in particular the crust, has gotten an undeserved reputation for being difficult to make or for the realm of expert bakers only. But like anything really worth having in life—the girl or boy of your dreams, a master's degree, playing in a band with your best friends—a modicum of commit- ment, dedication, and willingness to get stuff under your fingernails pays off big.

Paging though the book, it's apparent that our definition of "pie" is a generously pro- portioned net, scooping up unlikely items such as cheesecakes, cobblers, and even a pandowdy or a buckle. That's where the "ve- gan" in "pie in the sky" steps in. Compas- sionate desserts free of animal products are our trade, and we thought it only fair to in- clude anything that goes beyond the defini- tion of "cupcake" or "cookie" and typically requires baking in a pan of sorts. And be- cause you, dear vegan baker, need cheese- cakes, cream pies, dreamy whipped topping, and chocolate ganache-slicked tarts like the rest of the dessert-craving world.

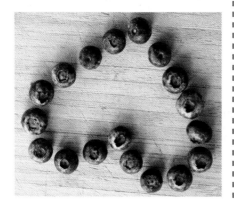

Like a good sense of humor or a little black dress, pie making will never be passé. Isn't it time for a slice of pie right now?

With love,

Terry and Isa

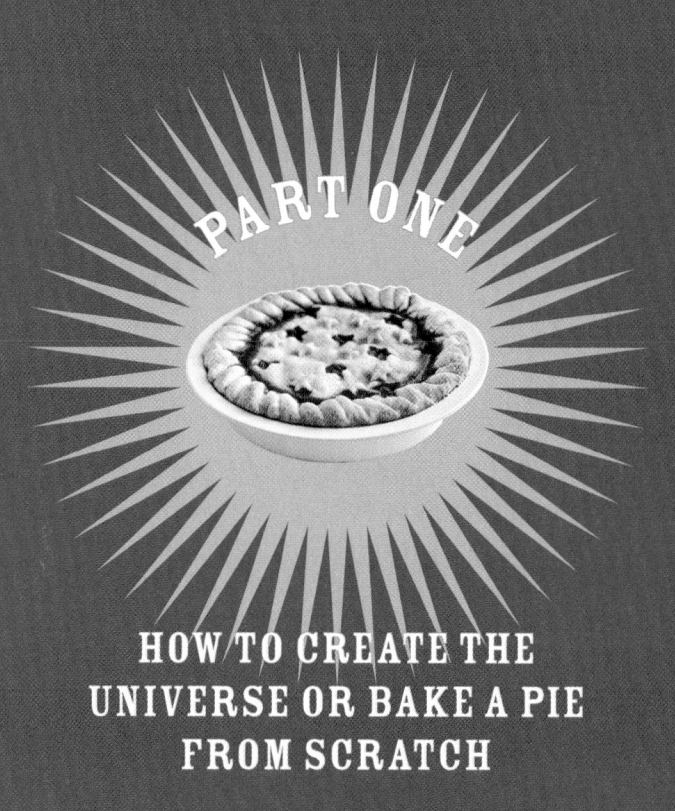

PART ONE

HOW TO CREATE THE UNIVERSE OR BAKE A PIE FROM SCRATCH

ESSENTIAL PIE INGREDIENTS

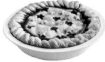

YOU ARE PROBABLY already familiar with apple, peaches, or pecans, but perhaps you could use a little guidance when it comes to the mysteries of agar powder, tapioca, or turbinado sugar. Vegan pie baking diverges only slightly from regular pie baking, but take the time to skim through this chapter before shopping for ingredients to make sure your pantry is prepared for a frenzy of vegan pie.

CREAMY THINGS

COCONUT MILK: Canned coconut milk will open a whole new world of rich, creamy, decadent, dairy-free desserts. Stick to full-fat coconut milk, not lite, for the recipes in this book. It's a small price to pay for vegan desserts that truly taste like a little slice of heaven.

CASHEWS: The nutty basis of so many creamy desserts in this book, cashews transform into creamy magic with an overnight soak in water and a fast puree in a blender. Alas, just as love shouldn't be complicated, neither should cashews, but somehow they both manage to be!

Here is the thing: You don't want *roasted* or *salted* cashews here. Roasted cashews have an assertive toasty taste that you don't want to overpower the other ingredients. And, unfortunately the term "raw" can be confusing. Some grocery stores mark their cashews as "raw" but they actually just mean "unroasted." And then there are "high raw" cashews that cost $17 a pound. Yikes! So if you see reasonably priced cashews marked "raw," grab 'em. But you can also use cashews simply marked "cashews." As long as the only ingredient is cashews and the package doesn't say "roasted" or "salted" or have any other adjective in front of it, you should be kosher. (Although it doesn't have to say "kosher" either.)

If you imagine yourself baking up scores of creamy pies and cheesecakes, run out right now and buy a great big bag of cashews. We promise you'll make good use of them in this book, even if it's just for making RAD WHIP (page 199) to smother fruit pies with.

½ cup whole raw cashews = 3.5 ounces

1 cup whole raw cashews = 7 ounces

SOY MILK, ALMOND MILK, AND OTHER NONDAIRY MILK FRIENDS: Almond, soy, hemp, oat, rice: It's all good when it comes to baking pies. Unlike most baking, with a few exceptions, the recipes in this book need only fairly small quantities of the stuff, so use what you like. We've gone ahead and made some suggestions in recipes, but ultimately follow your nondairy heart. Same goes for sweetened versus unsweetened milk as well.

TOFU: It wouldn't be a vegan cookbook without a little tofu talk, but breathe easy knowing that the only kind you need to know is silken tofu, the smooth and delicate tofu that makes luscious vegan cheesecakes, creams, and mousses a reality. If possible, look for fresh, water-packed tofu in the refrigerated section of your grocery, but if that's not possible, shelf-stable boxed Mori-Nu silken tofu is great, too.

FLOURS & STARCHES

ALL-PURPOSE FLOUR: All-purpose unbleached is just what the pie doctors ordered, but health nuts can substitute up to half the amount of flour in a recipe with white whole wheat flour with similar results. While we like whole wheat pastry flour for tender muffins and cookies, rolled pie dough needs the additional gluten that all-purpose flour provides. We use a few different flours in the book for fun, but APF is really all you need.

★ ★ ★

SO MANY THICKENERS, SO LITTLE TIME

WE GET ASKED this all the time, and maybe you're wondering, too: How do you decide which thickener to use? The answer really depends on your personal preference. Tapioca gives pie fillings a nice thick gooeyness. But it can sometimes be too gooey and too thick, so we will often temper it with other starches. All-purpose flour is also an old-school way to thicken fruit pies; it lends a creamy texture to apple pie filling we adore. Overall, cornstarch does a great job and is always consistent, so we gravitate toward that one the most.

CORNSTARCH: Good-old cornstarch is a cheap and reliable thickener of puddings, creams, and a cornucopia of other pie fillings. Always have a big box of cornstarch on hand whenever baking anything! We use exclusively organic to avoid that pesky GMO corn. Obviously, it's a bit more pricey and hard to find, so why not order a bunch of it online? Amazon.com has good deals all the time.

TAPIOCA: Tapioca flour or tapioca powder (same thing) is an old-fashioned pie-filling thickener, but there's no need to bother with tapioca pearls when tapioca flour is so readily available these days. Tapioca is sometimes used interchangeably with cornstarch in recipes, but we feel it does have a different kind of cooked texture (thicker, gooier), so proceed with caution. When we use it we reserve it for the occasional berry pie, but try both and see which you like best for thickening fruit pies.

ARROWROOT: This is a starch that comes from the root of an herb. We don't specifically call for arrowroot in our recipes, but if you are in love with this thickener, you can use it in place of cornstarch.

AGAR POWDER (AKA AGAR-AGAR): Vegan gelatin! Because seaweed is better than

ALL ABOUT AGAR

AGAR POWDER, also called agar-agar (like Duran Duran, it's one of those things that demands two names), is derived from a seaweed and is an absolutely essential ingredient for sophisticated vegan desserts. When boiled and melted into a liquid it has a powerful jelling ability, not unlike gelatin. But wait, it doesn't stop there! Agar powder not only is a substitute for gelatin, but also provides the same setting qualities that eggs and some dairy products do in traditional cooked custards and puddings, the basis for many creamy pie fillings.

If you've ever prepared a box of gelatin in your pre-vegan life, you can totally handle using powdered agar! Don't panic.

RULE ZERO ABOUT AGAR POWDER: WORK HOT AND WORK FAST!
Agar will continue to amaze you in that unlike stupid gelatin, agar will set as it cools no matter what the outside temperature is. It can even set at room temperature! That's right; if you cooked a batch of vanilla custard with agar powder, get a call from your best friend gushing about her new food processor, talk with her for three hours and forget your custard on the stove, don't fear. Agar did all the work while you gabbed, and it will be as firm and bouncy as if you did remember to put it in the fridge. That's the good news. The bad news is that means you must, absolutely must, work quickly when cooking with agar. Immediately after boiling, blend (if the recipe calls for it) and pour agar into a crust right away while it's still hot! Agar-agar waits for no man.

NOT THE SAME: AGAR POWDER VERSUS AGAR FLAKES
If only our mothers had told us to stay away from flakes. Agar flakes, that is. They technically may be the same as agar powder, but the powder cooks up smooth, melts fast,

ALL ABOUT AGAR (CONTINUED)

and is vastly consistent compared to its flaky cousin. As of this writing, unfortunately flakes are usually the only agar product most natural food stores carry and that sucks. Visit your local Asian grocery and seek out unsweetened packets of agar powder (make sure it's just agar without sugar or anything else added); the Thai brand Telephone is a favorite of ours and usually found for pennies. Buy plenty of it; when stored in a dry, cool place agar lasts nearly forever.

A LITTLE GOES A LONG, LONG WAY
Agar is powerful stuff and a little bit goes a long way. In general, for creamy pie fillings that need just a little extra help holding together, we like to use a ratio of 1 teaspoon of powder (remember, never flakes!) to 2½ cups of filling.

---

cow skin (yuck). This book uses exclusively the powdered kind, and because everyone asks, no, you cannot grind agar flakes into a powder. We use it to set creamy desserts and toppings. Check out "All About Agar" for more info on this magical substance.

SWEETENERS

This is a dessert cookbook after all, and sweeteners you must use. In the sea of sweeteners on store shelves these days we still rely on just a handful for consistent and dependable pie baking.

PLAIN OLD SUGAR: Cheap, easy to use, neutral in flavor and very reliable in results, it's still hard to beat sugar when making desserts. Vegan police: Because some cane sugars are filtered through animal bones, and you can't really know the refining process, you can always use beet sugar instead, or you can use evaporated cane juice or Florida Crystals. Whole Foods has a brand that they mark "Vegan Sugar," which is fine for most things, but we prefer the white stuff for caramel.

TURBINADO SUGAR: That big crystal '90s natural darling of coffee shops is fantastic for sprinkling on top of cobblers or top crusts for an extra sweet sparkle and crunch. We still prefer to use sugar for sweetening the inside of pies, so while not a necessity, it's worth picking up a small bag of turbinado just for sprinkling.

MAPLE SYRUP: Sometimes only maple-y goodness will do! In its pure form, it tends to be expensive, so we pair it with only a few pies, like MAPLE-KISSED BLUEBERRY PIE (page 57), MAPLE PECAN PIE (page 157), and the best pumpkin pie you've ever had (page 155).

FATS

Pie crusts need fat the way a fish needs a bicycle. Wait—we mean, the way a fish needs water. Fat provides the flavor, tender crumb, and delightful flake you came here for, so don't be shy when working fat into that pie dough.

SHORTENING & MARGARINE: The quintessentially American pie crust ingredient. By now most any natural foods store is home to nonhydrogenated, high-quality margarine. As of this writing, vegan Earth Balance is the best-tasting nonhydrogenated margarine available; look for it in stick form for super-convenient crust making.

OILS: Canola and even extra-virgin olive oil are both great alternatives to solid fats and are easy pantry-ready items. Go to the Pie Crust section (page 36) for recipes featuring these fats.

UNREFINED COCONUT OIL: We use coconut oil in many of our pies because it's solid at room temperature and great for giving mousses and cheesecakes stability while adding excellent creamy texture.

A FEW MORE STAPLES

FROZEN FRUIT: Since it can't always be summer, frozen fruit is the next best thing. Use only fruit that has been frozen loose and packed in bags. Definitely avoid frozen fruit that's processed with sugar or syrup and packed into unseemly blocks. For best results, avoid frozen fruit that is too old or has accumulated a lot of ice; it will ooze out too much water when thawed and baked. For pitch-perfect pies using frozen fruit, make sure to read our treatise "Two Frozen Berries Enter, One Cooked Berry Leaves: Tips for Using Frozen Fruit"on page 12.

★ ★ ★

THE FROZEN PIE CRUST QUESTION

WE UNDERSTAND THE SIREN SONG of frozen premade pie crusts: no rolling pin, no flour all over the kitchen (and the cat), no need to pinch dough edges into little shapes. If the ingredients are vegan and you need a pumpkin pie or crumb-topped fruit pie right now, it's hard to beat the convenience of a frozen crust. And, just in case you need it, we give you permission to use them!

You can also MacGyver a top crust with a frozen crust; this works best for chunky double-crust fruit pies like apple or peach (or purposely ragged-looking PANDOWDY, page 82). It's easy! Without removing the pan, flip the crust onto a sheet of waxed paper. Let thaw until the crust is soft and pliable, then lift up the pan to remove the crust; the crust may sink a little bit but don't worry about it, just gently press together any cracks.

To complete the pie, slide the crust on top of a filled bottom crust. Moisten your fingers and press out any cracks, slice a few vent holes on top, brush with soy milk, and sprinkle with sugar. This top crust may not win any beauty contest but sometimes you just gotta have pie and have it now, so bake immediately!

TWO FROZEN BERRIES ENTER, ONE COOKED BERRY LEAVES
TIPS FOR USING FROZEN FRUIT

IT'S THE MIDDLE OF JANUARY and you need homemade blueberry pie. *Now.* Well lucky you, today's frozen fruit is a world away from the syrupy, sloppy frozen fruit of the past. Many supermarkets and most natural food stores can supply anyone with top quality frozen berries–blueberries, blackberries, cherries, mixed berries–that will whisk your winter pies into mid-July. However there are a few tips to keep in mind for optimal baking results.

These tips mostly concern frozen berries, due to to the fact they're basically little sacks of ice and will break down during baking considerably more than fresh berries (hence the title). Sliced frozen peaches are less fussy; see tips for handling frozen peaches on page 66 for **BASIL PEACH PIE**.

❖ Use only loosely packed, unsweetened frozen berries sold in plastic bags. Never use berries frozen solid in sugar syrup.

❖ Keep berries frozen until ready to use. When ready to bake, quickly combine berries with other filling ingredients, top as directed in the recipe, and bake immediately in a preheated oven.

❖ Use a little more powdered thickener in the filling. Add an additional ¼ teaspoon to ½ teaspoon of cornstarch or tapioca flour per cup of frozen fruit. The more starch you add, the thicker the filling will be.

❖ Bake as directed for fruit pies, at 425°F for 20 minutes first, then reducing heat to 350°F, but you'll likely need to bake an additional 10–15 minutes. If your results are still a little too watery, consider turning down the heat to 400°F for the first part and bake for 30 minutes, then reduce heat to 350°F.

THE VODKA CRUST PHENOMENON

Hold onto your martinis; vodka isn't just for drinking anymore. The latest trend in pie crust (did you know there were crust trends?) is substituting chilled vodka for some of the ice water in crusts, resulting in even more flakiness. The science behind it claims that unlike water, the alcohol prevents the formation of gluten—the protein found in wheat flour. The end result is a lighter, flakier texture. While we prefer to keep our pie crusts straight and narrow, you may try your hand at using vodka for your own boozy crust adventures and see which is best for you.

We recommend using an inexpensive vodka (you won't taste it in the baked dough, so save the good stuff for after hours) as a variation on the BUTTERY DOUBLE CRUST (page 37) or the SINGLE (AND LOVING IT!) PASTRY CRUST (page 42) (see recipes for detailed instructions). The resulting dough may be somewhat stickier, so be sure to give the dough an extra long chill in the refrigerator and try rolling it between sheets of plastic; a huge ziptop freezer bag is sturdier than plastic wrap and will prevent the need to work additional flour into the dough (which will develop the gluten even more and waste a perfectly good martini).

APPLE CIDER VINEGAR: Our favorite, old-fashioned way to keep crusts from developing a bad attitude, too much gluten and getting tough.

PURE VANILLA EXTRACT: Get a huge bottle that will last you a lifetime. Or at least a few months. Always use the real stuff, fancy glass bottle not mandatory but it is usually a sign of quality.

LEMONS: We prefer fresh lemon juice, right from the lemon. If you absolutely can't get any, then bottled pure lemon juice (not from concentrate) will work in recipes where lemon is not the main ingredient. So for the LITTLE LEMON MOUSSE PIES (page 103), go fresh, but a few tablespoons of bottled in a strawberry pie never hurt anyone.

STORE-BOUGHT WHIPPED TOPPINGS

Vegan whipped toppings have come a long way from pureed tofu (thankfully!) If you are not inclined to make your own, there are a few that we can recommend out in the market today.

SOYATOO SOY WHIP (BOXED): A soy-based whipping cream that fluffs up nicely and tastes smooth and creamy. The same brand offers a spray can whipped topping, but we recommend the box for the most consistent and stable results. Found in the dairy section of your local Whole Foods.

MIMICCREME HEALTHY TOP: An almond- and cashew-based cream that has a rich, luscious flavor and texture. This one is shelf stable and usually found in the baking aisle, but it's worth buying online if you can't find it, since you won't have to pay an exorbitant rate for an ice pack (veganessentials.com).

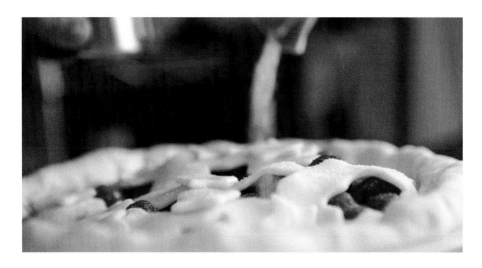

PIE-MAKING EQUIPMENT

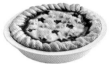

AS COMPLICATED as pie sometimes seems, the truth is that it can be blessedly simple. In fact, you can make a great pie with nothing but a fork, mixing bowl, and pie plate. You can even use a wine bottle as a rolling pin if you like! We've provided DIY solutions for the beginner pie maker, but the more intrepid among us might want to gather a few more tools for the ride.

ESSENTIALS

ROLLING PIN: Marble or wood, pick your poison! Isa prefers the American-style rolling pin with handles, but Terry is all about the French-style solid dowel pin.

DIY: Keep it real with a wine bottle, if you don't mind the dough getting a little uneven.

CRUST SHIELDS: Crust shields are great for those moments when the crust is saying "I'm ready" but the filling is saying "Let's wait." Slip on a pie crust shield and everything will bake in perfect harmony. Although we are not usually fans of silicon in baking, we really love the flexible silicon crust protector. (A tin one will also do just fine.) Some pie books may tell you to put the protectors on before baking, but we recommend placing them on halfway through baking to avoid crushing that pretty pie crust edge you labored over.

DIY: You can probably fashion a crust protector out of aluminum foil. It's not very fun, but it will work.

PIE WEIGHTS: The moisture in pastry crust creates steam and steam creates puffiness, which is great for flakiness, but not so great when you're parbaking a single pie crust. It can make the empty crust puff up so much that you can't fit enough filling—sadface! Pie weights to the rescue! These are ceramic, metal, or clay beads that keep that crust in place. You can place the weights directly onto the crust, but to make them easier to get out, place a round of parchment on the crust first.

DIY: Dried beans make awesome pie weights. Choose big beans like kidney or pinto.

PASTRY CUTTER (AKA PASTRY KNIFE): Depending on your own pie style (see the Pie Crusts chapter, page 36), you may want

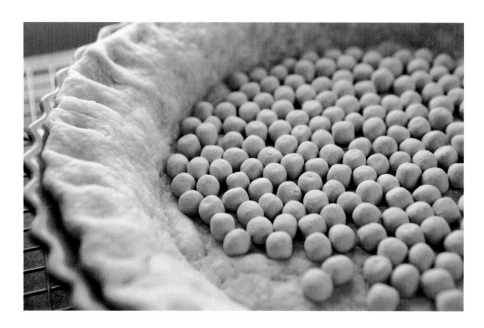

to add a pastry cutter to your baking arsenal. It cuts the fat into your flour like *whoa*, plus is a great way to take out your daily frustrations on pie crust.

DIY: You can hold two butter knives together to form a makeshift pastry cutter.

MIXING BOWLS: Truth: You can never have enough mixing bowls. We have about a zillion. But you should have at least three . . . a gigantic one, with plenty of space for tossing around flour and kneading dough, and two medium ones (preferably with a handle) for mixing berries and other fillings or beating together toppings. The convenience of extra mixing bowls is worth making extra dishes to wash.

RUBBER SPATULA: For scraping up the last remains of precious batter, topping, or filling and for smoothing out melted chocolate. A square-ended spatula is a champ at scraping out a food processor.

PANS

Most of the pies in this book require a 9-INCH PIE PAN. We suggest that you stock both a deep ceramic or Pyrex pie pan (about 2 inches deep) and a more shallow metal (or glass) pie pan. The deep pans are great for juicy fruit pies with glorious crimped pastry crusts and the shallow ones for sleek creamy pies with press-in cookie crusts. Note that deep-dish ceramic pans sometimes are closer to 10 inches wide, which is fantastic for juicy fruit pies and cobblers, so get one of these, too.

A 10-INCH FLUTED TART PAN with a removable bottom is essential for cream-filled or nutty tarts. We prefer the dark metal pans for crisp crusts. Tart pans with nonremovable bottoms work okay, but it's nearly impossible to get nice, clean slices out of them. Be easy on yourself and find that removable bottom!

We use 6 MINI (4-INCH) TART PANS with removable bottoms for a few recipes in the book. They can be great for making self-contained individual servings when you're feeling fancy.

A 9- TO 9½-INCH SPRINGFORM PAN is what you want for cheesecakes and mousse pies. Springform is pretty much a requirement here, since the sides just snap off, leaving you with a beautiful molded dessert that's a cinch to slice. Regular pie pans aren't the right shape, nor are they deep enough, so spring for a springform pan!

If you'd like to make mini-cheesecakes and mousse pies, these really cute desserts can be yours with a set of 3- to 4-inch MINI SPRINGFORM PANS.

DECORATING

COOKIE CUTOUTS: A few small, simple shapes can elevate your crusts from "Wow!" to a full-on, caps-lock "WOW!" For the best value, buy a whole team of adorable cutout shapes in a single package. Hearts, stars, diamonds, and clovers are all contenders for adorable crust cutouts. (See page 32 for how to do it.) To keep cutters from sticking to the dough while you're cutting out shapes, dip them occasionally in flour.

RAVIOLI WHEEL (AKA PASTRY WHEEL): For a pretty fringe on your lattice-top pies, or just to cut your pastry strips with preci-sion, a ravioli wheel may be just what the baker ordered. Bonus: You can use it to make ravioli!

DIY: A steak knife usually works just fine.

PASTRY BRUSH: Pie crusts brushed with a little soy milk and sprinkled with sugar make for an excellent crunchy texture and a sweet little surprise. You can use your fingertips to get the job done, but a pastry brush is just so much classier.

DIY: A silicon brush from a kitchen supply store is a serious baking tool, but a cheap and good option is a regular old 2-inch nylon paintbrush from a housewares store.

PASTRY BAG AND PASTRY TIPS: You can apply some of your cupcake panache to pie baking! Creamy pies beg to be decorated with swooping swirls of vegan whipped cream, or drizzled with chocolate. Have on hand a few pastry bags (plastic or waxed canvas) and some pastry tips: a tiny circle for drizzles, a large star tip for big florets, and a large circle tip for pretty clouds of cream.

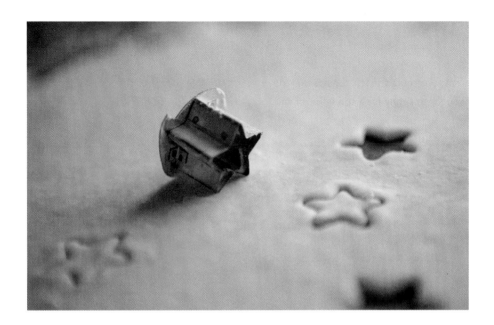

DIY: A large plastic ziptop bag with a half-inch slice snipped from the corner can give you surprisingly good piping results, too.

SMALL APPLIANCES

BLENDER OR FOOD PROCESSOR: You can easily get through this pie book without having one of those $400 crush-all-in-its-path techno blenders (like Blendtec or Vitamix). But you will definitely need a blender or food processor for creating creamy fillings. They also make quick work of cookies for crumb crusts. Some people also prefer a food processor for making their pie crusts (see page 25 for how it's done.)

HANDHELD ELECTRIC MIXER: We use a handheld mixer for only a few things: whipped toppings and the peanut butter filling. But isn't that reason enough?

MICROWAVE: We give! We give! We have finally realized that a microwave is the primo device for melting chocolate in small quantities. Culinary gods, forgive us.

AND DON'T FORGET!

OVEN THERMOMETER: As always, we insist that you have an oven thermometer for accuracy. Ovens are your enemy; they will lie, cheat, and steal in order to foul up your pastry plans. Never turn your back and always use an oven thermometer!

TIMER: In case you get lost in your *Buffy* marathon, always remember to set a timer to avoid sad-making burnt crusts and pouty-face overbaked cheesecakes. A well-mannered oven (even one that needs a thermometer) may come with a timer, so use it!

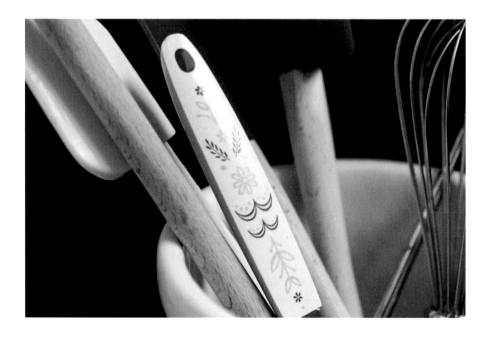

HOW TO SPY A PIE

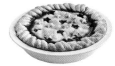

BETTY: A casserole almost always made with apples or pears layered with buttery breadcrumbs.

BUCKLE: Similar to a cobbler but more like a cake, here the fruit is piled on top of batter. As the cake batter bakes, it rises and buckles around the fruit.

COBBLER: What makes a cobbler a cobbler is the top crust: It should be batter- or biscuit-like and nice and thick.

CRISP: Again, it's all about the topping. A crisp has a crumbly topping, usually oats, flour, nuts, or some combination thereof.

GALETTE: A free-form tart. Also called a crostada, and often evoking the word "rustic."

HAND PIE: Sure, you could pick up a whole pie and eat it with your hands. But a hand pie is a tiny pie designed to do so!

PIE: You know what a pie is. A crust, a filling, and a topping. Of course we play with the definition a bit, but that's the gist. The topping for a pie can be a rolled-out pastry, a crumble, or a lattice. We don't discriminate!

PANDOWDY: Bake a pie halfway through, then smash the top crust into the filling and continue to bake, and you've got pan-dowdy. Why do this? Surely it started as a mistake somewhere. But the gooey results are delicious.

TART: Loosely defined, it's a pie with no top. But it's also generally a thinner, sleeker affair, pressed into a wide, shallow tart pan.

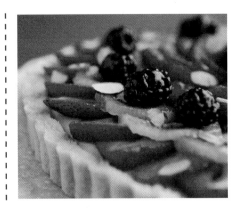

ROLL WITH IT
Making Great Homemade Pie Crust

HOMEMADE PIES CRUSTS are like thumbprints; no two are exactly the same. Both of us (Isa and Terry here) have different methods, and maybe you already have a method that you love. There's only one pie crust rule of thumb (no pun intended): Practice, practice, and when you're all done, practice some more!

The first pie crust you'll ever make may range from acceptable to something resembling a feral pancake, but no worries. The second one will be better, the third beyond better, the fourth something to blog about, and so on. Don't be afraid to get some flour on your apron, roll up your sleeves, and let yourself relax and enjoy the feeling of the rolling pin gliding across the dough. It's pie dough, not rocket science, so it's okay to make mistakes.

HOW TO MAKE PIE CRUST, STEP BY STEP

Most pie crusts are basically the same concept: starchy flour melded with ample fat for flavor and texture, plus a little bit of liquid to help hold everything together. There are a few exceptions in regards to the addition of liquid, but beyond that a pie crust is a rich pastry designed to hold in soft, wet fillings.

Your basic pie crust starts its life as a bowl of flour and a little salt. The next step is to blend a fat—cold margarine, chilled shortening, or even cold oil—into the flour. There are a few ways to do this that work equally well, and both of us have our favorite method. If you don't already have a preferred method, try a few and see for yourself!

So why bother with adding fat in crusts? Fat does a double duty in pie crust: It ensures that the gluten (the protein in wheat flour that gives baked goods structure) doesn't become stretchy, keeping the gluten strands short (thus the word *shortbread* for the kind of dough that is just flour, fat, and sugar). Keeping the fats cold creates steam pockets when the crust hits the heat, resulting in a light, flaky dough. It also provides the rich, smooth flavor, crispness, and melt-in-your-mouth quality you're looking for in a well-made crust.

STEP 1: *Work in the fat*

After stirring together dry ingredients in a large mixing bowl, drop in tablespoons of cold fat, in the form of tablespoons of margarine, shortening, or oil.

Now quickly cut the fat into the dough. The method for pastry dough is a bit different than for other forms of baking. Unlike mix-ing a muffin batter or cookie dough, here you're not mixing things together. Rather, you're cutting the fat into the flour, keeping the fat intact but still getting it well distributed throughout the final pastry, so the end result looks a little like cornmeal or polenta meal. Here's where you have options!

There are a few different ways to blend the fat into the flour. Isa likes to use her fingertips. With this method, add half of the fat called for at first, in about half-tablespoon-size chunks. Rub the fat into the flour with your fingertips until it gets pebbly. Then add the remaining fat and again, continue to rub it into the flour. Doing it in two sessions like that distributes smaller and bigger pieces of fat, which makes a tender and flaky crust.

If you are a fan of kitchen gadgets, then you'll like Terry's preferred method of using a pastry cutter. A quick internet search will reveal something that looks like a series of thin metal loops curved around a handle. It's an affordable utensil that makes quick work of cutting fat into flour, while giving you a satisfying punching-bag-style work-out. It also helps keep the fat a little colder by limiting exposure to melting heat from one's hands, handy if you're making pastry on a hot summer day or in hell. Work in the fat, rocking the pastry cutter against the bottom of the mixing bowl and turning the bowl a few degrees occasionally until you have a pebbly mixture.

STEP 2: *Add water and acid*

Basic pie dough needs a little liquid, usually water, to help pull it together. The trick is to approach it the way Goldilocks would make pie dough: not too much, not too little, just the right amount of liquid. So really we want the pie dough to have as little water as possible, but we still need a little bit so that the dough is pliable and easy to roll.

This is done by drizzling ice water into the crust by the tablespoon, gently mixing it in with your fingertips or a rubber spatula. The crust is ready to be formed into a ball when you can squeeze a clump in your hand and have it hold together. If needed, drizzle in up to two more tablespoons and try again.

The finished dough should want to stick together and easily form a ball; it should not be sticky or wet, nor crumbly and sandy. If you're just starting out making pie dough

★ ★ ★

PASTRY OUT OF A FOOD PROCESSOR

IN ADDITION TO BARE HANDS and using a pastry cutter, food processors have become a popular third option for making fast, smooth pie pastry. If you have a large food processor with a big cutting blade then you'll soon be in the business of making speedy pastry. Simply whirl together the dry ingredients, then add a chunk of fat at a time, pulsing until an evenly crumbly mixture is achieved. Now slowly drizzle in the minimal amount of liquid into the neck of the food processor. The dough is ready when it gathers into a ball and away from the sides of the food processor bowl. It can take mere seconds to mix up dough this way, so be careful not to overwork the dough!

you're probably better off erring on the side of a slightly moist dough that won't break apart during rolling, but as you make more crusts you'll be able to identify that sweet spot of moisture content of a well-made dough.

You'll also notice that we use a touch of apple cider vinegar in many of the crust recipes. Acidity is another thing that keeps crusts tender by making sure that the gluten doesn't develop and toughen the crust. Don't worry about the vinegar smell; it bakes out of the crust and you'll never guess it was ever there.

STEP 3: *Divide and chill*
Divide the dough in two (if doing a double crust; if it's a single crust, don't bother), lightly knead each piece into a ball, and then pat it into a disk about an inch thick. Wrap the dough in plastic wrap and refrigerate for a minimum of half an hour. Chilling the dough helps further tame that gluten, making it easier to roll. If you do refrigerate the dough overnight, just let it sit out for about 10 minutes or until it's just soft enough to roll.

Tightly wrapped dough can last up to a week in the refrigerator. Just try to avoid getting the dough soggy with condensation from too many days in the cold; this will toughen your dough and ruin the flavor.

If you really need to freeze pie dough (we'd rather you make a batch at a time when needed), chill it, roll it out flat and layer it between waxed paper. Store in big, tightly sealed freezer bags, and when you're ready to use it, let it thaw on a kitchen counter until it's soft and pliable. Another way to freeze crust is to press it into the pie plate you intend on baking it in and just go ahead and freeze.

STEP 4: *Roll 'em out*
To roll the crust, first make sure you have loads of space! This is of utmost importance. You need plenty of elbow room, so if your counter space is cramped, try the kitchen table. It's also easiest to roll out dough if you use your body weight, instead of straining your hands and wrists. You want to lean into it. So it's best if you're standing, because sitting just won't get you the pressure you need.

A clean, dry, lightly floured, cool surface is the most versatile place to roll out pie dough. A marble or granite countertop is just about perfect, but a really big smooth cutting board works equally well.

If you don't want to be bothered with messing up the countertop, you can roll dough between sheets of waxed paper liberally sprinkled with flour. Even better, sheets of thicker kitchen plastic (as in huge freezer bags) won't require the addition of flour. This is convenient, too, if you want to roll your dough but not fit it into a pie plate just yet; you can roll and store it covered with waxed paper in the fridge until ready to use.

Have a hot, steamy kitchen? If you're baking in the middle of the summer berry season without air conditioning it's bound to happen, so consider getting all of your crust-making equipment as cold as possible. So go ahead and throw that rolling pin in the fridge while your dough chills. Give it a wipe if any moisture condenses on it.

Enough chatter, let's get to rolling!

Instead of dusting the rolling pin with flour, just lightly dust the top of the pie dough. Roll from the center out, in all directions, occasionally rotating the dough a few degrees after each pass with the rolling pin. Lightly dust with flour and carefully flip the dough over once, and then roll it out the rest of the way, to 12 or 13 inches. The edges may be a little frazzled and crumbly, and that is just great! This means that the dough is not overworked. But it shouldn't be completely cracking and turning into a lopsided amoeba, either. If that happens, let it rest a bit more at room temp and gently cut away any "arms" of the amoeba and press them into other edges of the dough, roll to seal and to reshape everything back into roughly a circle. The finished dough should be about ¼ inch thick, maybe a tiny bit thicker for bottom crusts.

Once rolled out, gently lift your dough into the pie plate. If the pie pan is right there (and if not, why isn't it?), you shouldn't have a problem just plopping it in. It's as easy as sliding your hand underneath the center of the dough circle (if necessary, gently lift it around the edges first to unstick it from the rolling surface) and quickly flipping it into the pan.

Or try a less acrobatic method: Loosely roll about half of the dough back around the rolling pin, lift it over the pie plate, and unroll it. Gently press the dough into the plate and smooth out any wrinkles around the edges from the overlapping dough.

Finally, use a sharp kitchen scissors to trim the dough evenly so that you have about 1½ to 2 inches of dough hanging down from the edge of the plate. Now you're ready to crimp the edges!

PIE CRUST EDGES

There's a whole world of methods to seal the edges of your hard-earned pie crust, but for simplicity and ease, you really need only a few clever techniques. Try them all and figure out what your signature crimp will be, or just throw everyone off and use a different crimp every time.

Here are a few of our favorite methods for creating pretty and functional crust edges.

They're easy! General rule of thumb (no pun intended yet), fold any overhanging dough under so it's now sitting just on the edge of the plate before committing any crimping acts.

PINCHED FLUTE: Your fingers make great pie sealers. Using your thumb and forefinger, pinch the edges of the dough to resemble a wavy fluted shape all around the edges of the pie.

LARGE FLUTED SCALLOPED: Just like its little cousin the pinched flute, but mold the dough around the knuckle of your forefinger while pressing around it with your thumbs. Makes a big wavy edge around the pie.

FORK: Press the tines of a dinner fork into the pie edge. Depending on the angle or overlapping of marks, you can get a few interesting effects with just a plain old fork!

SPOON: Another amazing pie gadget that doubles as an eating utensil, spoon indentations are lovely and dainty on an otherwise flat and boring pie edge.

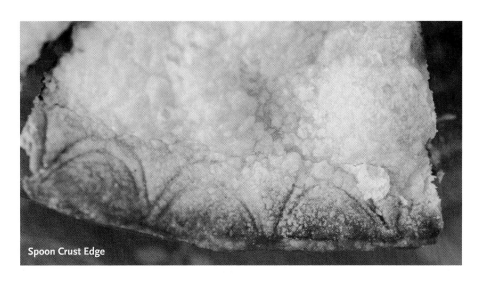

Spoon Crust Edge

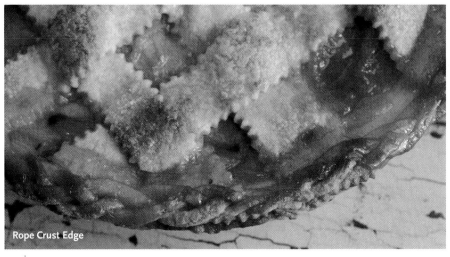

Rope Crust Edge

ROPE: A great use for leftover dough scraps and super elegant too! Gather and roll scraps into a long, 14-inch rectangle a little less than an inch wide. Trim the edges evenly and then slice it in half lengthwise, exactly down the center. Braid together the two long pieces of dough. Brush the flattened edge of your crust with soy milk and gently press the braid in, trimming any excess and taking care not to crush the braid design.

BUTTER KNIFE: Instead of just folding the overhanging edge, roll the excess crust inward, so it's a plump roll around the edges of the crust. Use a butter knife to press in slashes at a diagonal around the pie.

See SHE'S MY CHERRY PIE on the cover and on page 55 for an example of this edge.

PLAIN OLD FLAT SEAL VS. FANCY DOUGH CUTOUTS: Exactly what it sounds like, to create a flat seal just gently press down the folded edge of the dough. Maybe a little too plain? Dress it up with tiny cutouts using leftover dough; little shapes like hearts or leaves or stars look best.

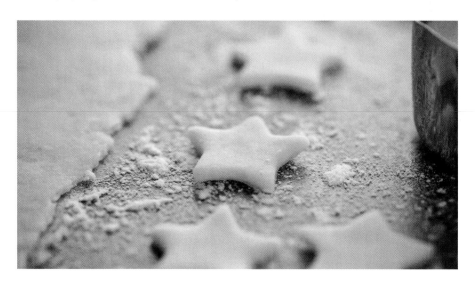

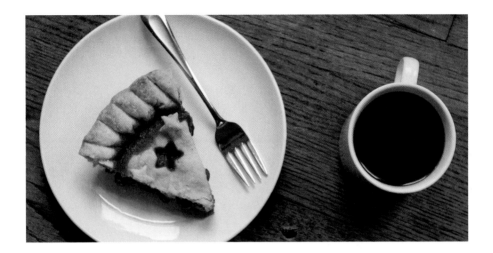

Brush these with water or soy milk to help seal them onto the dough.

PIE TOPS

First impressions often mean everything, pie upper crusts included. We have our own preferences (slitted blankets for apple, lattices for berry pies), but try any of these on your favorite fillings and see if they make a difference.

SIMPLY SLIT: A blanket of dough looks nice, but at minimum your pie needs a few slits to help steam escape during a pie's long baking process. A circle of five to six slits done in a radial pattern in the center of the top crust is all it takes to make a truly honest-looking crust. Especially pleasing on apple pies.

CUT-INS: Where cookie baking and pie crust meet! Roll out the top crust as directed, but use small, 1-inch wide cookie cutters to cut patterns into the top crust. Randomly or with purpose, a few hearts or leaves or moons or stars can make an ordinary crust extraordinarily adorable. Work

> ### ★ ★ ★
> ### SHOOT TO CHILL
>
> Unbaked pie crust loves to be cold, and a second chilling *after* you've pressed and
> crimped it into the pie plate is a good idea to help reduce shrinking and buckling of
> the dough as it bakes. We find this especially helpful for single-crust pies, where the
> crimped edge often serves as a focal point of decoration. Try chilling the crust for at
> least 30 minutes or preferably an hour before blind baking or full baking; it should help
> preserve your crimp artistry.

fast and don't let the dough get too warm, as the shapes may stretch and get distorted when moving a too-warm crust onto the pie.

CUTOUTS: Like cut-ins, except use a larger cutter, 2 to 2½ inches, and cut out enough shapes to completely cover the top of the pie for an elaborately layered look. Gently brush the edges of the cut outs with water or nondairy milk and layer over the pie, gently pressing together occasionally but taking care to preserve the shapes. When done brush everything again and sprinkle with sugar before baking.

LATTICE: This woven pie top screams "I am a domestic warrior!," looks super homespun yet classy, and is deceptively simple to achieve. Consult our handy illustration (opposite) because it's easier shown than explained! Try cutting the dough with a wavy-edged pastry wheel for an extra touch of grandma-worthy charm.

LAZY LATTICE: A lattice for the weekend pie maker or just the full-time lazy. Instead of weaving the dough strips, place strips in an evenly spaced layer over the pie, and then top with another evenly spaced layer of strips arranged perpendicular to the bottom strips.

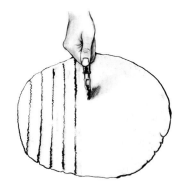

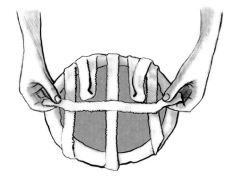

1. Roll out top crust to about ¼-inch thickness. Slice into ¾ to 1 inch wide parallel strips (use a ruler to help guide cutting) with either a sharp knife or pastry wheel.

2. Arrange strips on top of filled pie; use longest strip for the center. Leave space between strips equal to the thickness of the strips. Working from the center long strip, gently fold back every other strip and place another long strip parallel in the center of the pie.

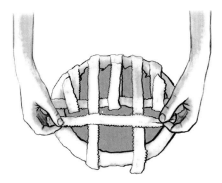

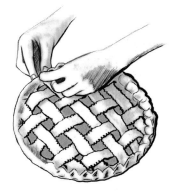

3. Unfold these strips over the parallel strip. Now fold back the strips not previously used and place another parallel strip; repeat as directed to weave strips of dough, working one side of the pie. Do the same on the other side of the pie, gently folding, arranging and unfolding strips.

4. When lattice is assembled, roll up hanging edges of bottom crust and fold over ends of dough strips. Crimp edges as desired and bake as directed.

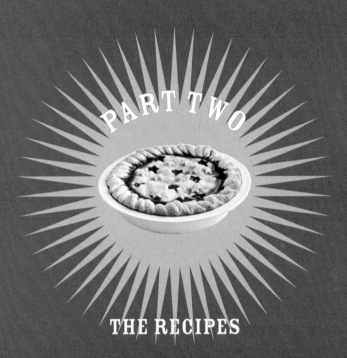

PART TWO

THE RECIPES

PIE CRUSTS

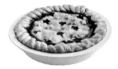

THAT CRISP, FLAKY, GOLDEN, crimped or fluted crust is what says pie to us, you, your grandmother, and the guy walking his dog outside the window as we type this. Fully cooled or piping hot, it's what gets nibbled first (or set aside to be savored last) by the die-hard pie crust aficionado.

If you've never rolled a crust from scratch, or did it once and swore you would never again, we want to bring you back into the pie-baking fold to try your hand at making a homemade crust. Made with high-quality vegan butter, shortening, or even olive oil, it's a taste that can't compare to anything store-bought.

BUTTERY DOUBLE CRUST

MAKES ONE 9-INCH TOP AND BOTTOM CRUST

THIS IS AN ALL-PURPOSE, flaky, roll-out pie crust, perfect for any of the pies in the book. It's great for cutting shapes, or making lattices.

2½ cups all-purpose flour

½ teaspoon salt

3 tablespoons sugar

8 tablespoons cold nonhydrogenated margarine

8 tablespoons cold nonhydrogenated shortening

6 tablespoons ice water

1 tablespoon apple cider vinegar

1. In a large mixing bowl, sift together the flour and salt. Mix in the sugar. Add half the margarine and shortening by about half tablespoonfuls, cutting it into the flour with your fingers or a pastry cutter, until the flour appears pebbly. Add the remaining margarine and shortening, and cut it into the flour.

2. In a cup, mix together 4 tablespoons of the ice water with the apple cider vinegar. Drizzle the water and vinegar mixture into the flour by the tablespoonful, gently mixing it after each addition. Knead the dough a few times, adding more water until it holds together. You may need only the 4 tablespoons, but add up to 2 more tablespoons if needed.

3. Divide the dough in two, roll each half into a ball, then press them into disks and wrap each in plastic wrap. Refrigerate them until ready to use, or use as directed in the recipe.

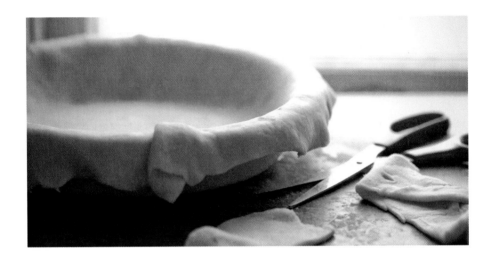

Variation

VODKA DOUGH: Say you want to be part of the vodka pie crust revolution (see page 13 for the benefits of a boozy dough). Start by sprinkling 4 tablespoons of inexpensive vodka over the flour mixture, then sprinkle on the apple cider vinegar. Gently stir a few times. Sprinkle in 4 tablespoons of water, a tablespoon at a time. Stir just enough to combine and gather the dough into a ball. If the dough is too crumbly, stir in more water, a tablespoon at a time, until the dough comes together but is not sticky. Proceed as directed.

Slices

An easy way to keep ice water handy is to plop a few ice cubes in a measuring cup of water. Just dip a tablespoon in as needed, then sprinkle into the dough.

OLIVE OIL DOUBLE CRUST

MAKES ONE 9-INCH TOP AND BOTTOM CRUST

THIS HAS BECOME OUR GO-TO CRUST. Olive oil produces a light, flaky crust with a surprisingly neutral taste. Plus, since it's made with pantry-friendly olive oil, it's a fast and convenient all-purpose crust ideal for fruit pies. The secret is to place the olive oil in the freezer beforehand, so that it becomes partially solid. This helps the fat blend into the dough in little pockets, creating the flakiness you crave.

2½ cups all-purpose flour

¾ teaspoon salt

⅔ cup olive oil, partially frozen (see instructions below)

4 to 8 tablespoons ice water

1 tablespoon apple cider vinegar

TO PREPARE THE OLIVE OIL:

1. About an hour before beginning the recipe, place the olive oil in a plastic container. For best results, use a thin, light container, like the kind used for takeout food. Freeze the oil until it's opaque and congealed but still somewhat soft, like the consistency of slightly melted sorbet. If it's over-frozen, that's okay; just let it thaw a bit so that you can work with it.

2. In a large mixing bowl, sift together the flour and salt. Working quickly, add the olive oil by the tablespoonful, cutting it into the flour with your fingers or a pastry cutter, until the flour appears pebbly.

3. In a cup, mix together 4 tablespoons of the ice water with the apple cider vinegar. Drizzle 2 tablespoons of the water and vinegar mixture into the dough and stir, using a wooden spoon or rubber spatula. Add more water, a tablespoon at a time, until the

dough holds together to form a soft ball. Take care not to over-knead the dough.

4. Divide the dough in two. Press each half into a disk about an inch thick and place each disk between two 14-inch long pieces of waxed paper. Using a rolling pin, roll each piece into a circle about ¼ inch thick. For a more even, uniform circle of dough, roll the pin one or two strokes outward, turn the dough a few degrees, and roll a few times again and repeat. Repeat with the other half of the dough. Refrigerate the rolled dough wrapped in waxed paper until it's ready to use, or as directed in the recipe.

ALL ABOUT COCONUT OIL CRUSTS

"Extra virgin," minimally processed coconut oil is now a mainstay in many natural foods kitchens. It is an ideal fat for a light, tender crust with a delicate coconut aroma. Since so many of our pie fillings use coconut milk or oil, we like to reserve coconut oil crusts for special occasions, but don't let that stop you from making any crust into a coconut oil crust sensation.

To use coconut oil in crusts, select an oil that's high quality and use when it's semisolid; coconut oil at a cool room temperature that is solid but easy to scoop with a measuring spoon. Use as directed in any recipe that calls for shortening, margarine, or canola oil.

PUFFY PIE DOUGH

MAKES ENOUGH DOUGH FOR 8 HAND PIES OR 2 FREE-FORM PIES

THIS DOUGH WITH A HINT of yogurt tartness isn't wildly puffy, like puff pastry, but bakes up puffier than the BUTTERY DOUBLE CRUST (page 37). It's the perfect dough for hand pies, because although the crust is sturdy enough to hold in juicy hand pie fillings, it's still tender to the bite.

2¼ cups all-purpose flour

3 tablespoons sugar

½ teaspoon salt

½ teaspoon baking powder

½ cup cold nonhydrogenated margarine

½ cup cold plain soy yogurt

¼ cup cold unsweetened nondairy milk

1. Sift the flour into a large mixing bowl, along with the sugar, salt, and baking powder. Add the margarine in about tablespoon-size pieces. Cut it into the flour with either a pastry cutter or your fingers.

2. Add half of the yogurt and mix, then add the remaining yogurt and mix. The dough should be clumpy. Add the milk and knead the mixture a few times with the heel of your hands, until a stiff dough forms.

3. Divide the dough in two, roll each piece into a ball and flatten them into disks. Wrap each in plastic wrap and chill them for 30 to 45 minutes, or until ready to use, or use according to the recipe directions.

SINGLE (AND LOVING IT!) PASTRY CRUST

MAKES ONE 9-INCH PASTRY BOTTOM CRUST

WHO SAYS IT TAKES TWO TO TANGO? This single crust is an all-American shortening-based pastry that's ready and willing for all of your bottom crust needs. It's a multitasker—this crust suits most any pie filling, creamy, fruity, and everything in between. For a richer flavor, substitute a high-quality vegan margarine for half of the shortening.

1½ cups all-purpose flour

2 tablespoons sugar

½ teaspoon salt

½ cup cold nonhydrogenated shortening

4 tablespoons or more ice water

2 teaspoons apple cider vinegar

1. Sift together the flour, sugar, and salt. Cut in the shortening (using forks; pastry cutter; fingers; food processor; robot slaves) to form a crumbly dough.

2. Stir together 4 tablespoons of the ice water and vinegar, then drizzle a third of it over the flour. Gently mix to moisten, drizzle in another third of the liquid, and mix to moisten. Repeat with the remaining mixture until the dough forms a soft ball when pressed together. If it hasn't come together yet, sprinkle it with another tablespoon (or more) of ice water until the dough can be gathered into a ball. Wrap it in plastic wrap or sandwich between waxed paper and refrigerate for an hour.

3. When you're ready to roll out the crust, tear off a 14-inch piece of waxed paper or baking parchment and lightly sprinkle it with flour. Flatten the dough into a disk and place it in the center of the paper. Using a lightly floured rolling pin in long, even strokes, roll out the

VEGAN PIE IN THE SKY

dough into a circle about 12 inches in diameter. Occasionally rotate the dough while you're rolling to help form an even circle.

4. To transfer the dough to a pie plate, slide your hand underneath the center of the paper and quickly flip it onto the plate. Peel off the paper and gently press the dough into the plate; if necessary, trim any overhanging dough edges with a sharp knife, leaving about 1½ inches of dough for the crimped edge. Crimp the edges as desired.

Slices

Try replacing
2 tablespoons of water with
an inexpensive vodka for a flakier crust.
See **BUTTERY DOUBLE CRUST**
recipe variation (page 38)
and page 13 for more
information.

SHORTBREAD TART SHELL

FILLS A 9- OR 10-INCH TART PAN OR SIX 4-INCH TART SHELLS

BUTTERY AND DELICATE yet surprisingly sturdy, this recipe is simple as can be to make, but follow the directions to ensure that your tart doesn't buckle and shrink when you prebake it. The secret isn't ours; any professional baking book will tell you that if you freeze the whole pan before baking, that will prevent shrinkage and the need for pie weights. Ample amount of fork pricks also help, so take that fork and go psycho on your crust.

1½ cups all-purpose flour

⅓ cup confectioner's sugar

⅛ teaspoon salt

¾ cup nonhydrogenated margarine

1. In a large mixing bowl, sift together the flour, sugar, and salt. Add the margarine in about tablespoon-size pieces. Cut the margarine into the flour with a pastry cutter or your fingers. Mix until the dough comes together.

2. Firmly press the dough into the tart pan(s). This works best if you first press and shape the sides of the crust and then press in the bottom. Using a fork, pierce the bottom and sides of the crust at even intervals, about 25 to 30 times. Freeze the crust for 45 minutes.

3. Once your crust is completely frozen, preheat the oven to 350°F. Bake for 10 minutes. Rotate the crust so that it cooks evenly and bake for another 15 minutes, or until lightly golden brown. Remove the crust from the oven and let it cool completely until it's ready to fill.

CHOCOLATE SHORTBREAD TART SHELL

FILLS A 9- OR 10-INCH TART PAN OR SIX 4-INCH TART SHELLS

A TENDER AND DEEPLY COCOA-FLAVORED variation of our favorite buttery shortbread shell. Because there's always more room for chocolate.

1 cup all-purpose flour

½ cup sifted cocoa powder

½ cup confectioner's sugar

⅛ teaspoon salt

¾ cup nonhydrogenated margarine

1. In a large mixing bowl, sift together the flour, cocoa powder, sugar, and salt. Add the margarine in about tablespoon-size pieces. Cut the margarine into the flour with a pastry cutter or your fingers. Mix until the dough comes together.

2. Firmly press the dough into the tart pan(s). This works best if you first press and shape the sides of the crust and then press in the bottom. Using a fork, pierce the bottom and sides of the crust at even intervals, about 25 to 30 times. Freeze the crust for 45 minutes.

3. Once your crust is completely frozen, preheat the oven to 350°F. Bake for 10 minutes. Rotate the crust so that it cooks evenly and bake for another 15 minutes, or until lightly golden brown. Remove the crust from the oven and let it cool completely until it's ready to fill.

GRAHAM CRACKER CRUST

IT'S HARD TO IMAGINE a mint chocolate pie, homespun pudding pie, or cheesecake without a sweet, crumbling crust made from crushed graham crackers, chocolate cookies, or even vegan vanilla wafers. Use this recipe for a firm crust that's ideal for slicing and holding in very soft pie fillings.

1¾ cups finely ground graham crackers (made from 10 ounces of whole graham crackers)

3 tablespoons sugar

4 tablespoons melted nonhydrogenated margarine, melted coconut oil, or canola oil

1 tablespoon plain soy milk or almond milk

1. Preheat the oven to 350°F and lightly spray a 9-inch pie plate with nonstick cooking spray.
2. In a mixing bowl, combine the graham crumbs and sugar. Drizzle in the oil or melted margarine. Use a spoon to blend the mixture thoroughly to moisten the crumbs, then drizzle in the soy milk and stir again to form a crumbly dough.
3. Pour the crumbs into the pie plate. Press crumbs into the sides of the plate first, then work your way down to the bottom. Bake for 8 to 10 minutes until firm. Let the crust cool before filling.

Variations

CHOCOLATE COOKIE CRUST: For a chocolate cookie crust, use ground-up vegan chocolate wafer cookies; a few natural food store brands (that are vegan as of this writing) we like are Mi-Del Chocolate Snaps and Newman's Own Chocolate Alphabet Cookies.

LEMON COOKIE CRUST: Mi-Del also makes regular and gluten-free Lemon Snaps. We love lemon crusts paired with the BLUEBERRY BLISS CHEESECAKE (page 95).

VANILLA COOKIE CRUST: For a vanilla cookie crust, use ground-up vegan vanilla wafers. We like the Back to Nature Madagascar Vanilla Wafers. Mi-Del also makes Vanilla Snap cookies.

BLACK & WHITE CRUST: For a Black & White crust, use equal portions of vanilla and chocolate cookie crumbs.

Slices

To pound down stubborn cookies, place them in a ziptop plastic bag, press out the air and seal. Use a rolling pin to crush them as finely as possible. You can use a food processor to create really fine cookie crumbs for a very evenly textured crust.

★ ★ ★

COOKIE CRUSTS FOR SPRINGFORM PANS

USE THE FOLLOWING amounts if you're baking up a cheesecake or making a mousse pie in a 9½-inch springform pan. Our testers found that springforms need a little less crust than pie plates; this is just the right proportion for a thin crust, patted only into the bottom of a springform pan.

1¼ cups finely ground graham cracker or chocolate cookie crumbs
3 tablespoons sugar
4 tablespoons melted nonhydrogenated margarine or coconut or canola oil
1 tablespoon soy milk

1. Prepare according to GRAHAM CRACKER CRUST (page 46) directions.

GINGERSNAP CRUST

SWEET AND SPICY, we adore this kicky crust paired with citrus fillings, creamy coconut fillings, or especially the CHAI-SPICED RICE PUDDING PIE (page 120). For use with cheesecakes (PUMPKIN CHEESECAKE [page 149] calling!), use the proportions listed in the tip box on page 47. We like using Mi-Del brand vegan gingersnaps, which as of this writing are also available gluten-free.

1¾ cups (about 10 ounces) vegan
gingersnap cookies
2 tablespoons brown sugar
4 tablespoons canola oil

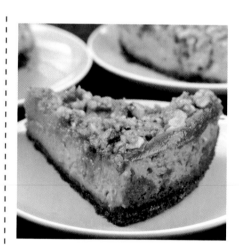

1. Grind the cookies into fine crumbs in a blender or food processor. Transfer the cookie crumbs to a mixing bowl and toss them together with the sugar and canola oil. The crust mixture is now ready to be pressed into a pie plate.

CHOCOLATE OLIVE OIL SHORTBREAD CRUST

FILLS A 9- OR 10-INCH TART PAN OR SIX 3- OR 4-INCH TART SHELLS

OLIVE OIL ADDS RICH, BUTTERY UNDERTONES to this crust that's essentially a great big chocolate cookie. The olive oil flavor works especially well with creamy fillings such as those used in the CHOCOLATE-ORANGE HAZELNUT TARTS (page 176), or encasing the LUXURY PISTACHIO PUDDING PIE (page 105).

1½ cups all-purpose flour

⅓ cup unsweetened cocoa powder

⅔ cup confectioner's sugar

¼ teaspoon salt

½ cup olive oil, partially frozen (see instructions in **OLIVE OIL DOUBLE CRUST**, page 39)

3 to 4 tablespoons almond milk

1. To make the dough, sift the flour, cocoa, and sugar together in a mixing bowl. Don't skip this step; you really need to break up the clumps. Rub the salt between your fingers to grind it down a little more, and add it to the mixture.

2. Add the olive oil to the flour mixture in tablespoonfuls. Use about ¼ cup at first, and cut it into the flour using either your fingers or a pastry cutter. Add the rest and keep cutting it in until the dough appears moist, clumpy, and crumbly. Drizzle in the almond milk (start with 3 tablespoons) and mix until the dough holds together when squeezed between your fingers.

3. Lightly spray the tart pan(s) with cooking spray. Distribute handfuls of dough equally amongst the pans if making multiple tarts, or pour all of it into a single pan. Firmly press the dough into the sides and bottom of the tart pan.

Now poke the shells all over with a fork and place in the freezer for about 30 minutes or until frozen solid.

4. Preheat the oven to 350°F. Take the tarts out of the freezer and place them on a large, rimmed baking sheet. Bake for 18 minutes, then remove from the oven and let cool. Once the crusts are cool enough to touch, they are ready to be filled.

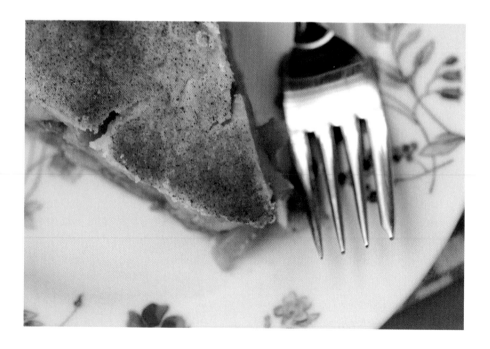

BUCKWHEAT DOUBLE CRUST

BUCKWHEAT ADDS A sultry yet homey flavor to dough. We love the rustic flair of a buckwheat crust, making this the perfect choice for free-form tarts and galettes.

1⅓ cups all-purpose flour

⅔ cup buckwheat flour

1 tablespoon sugar

½ teaspoon salt

½ cup cold, nonhydrogenated margarine

3 to 5 tablespoons ice water

1 tablespoon apple cider vinegar

1. In a large mixing bowl, sift together the flours, sugar, and salt. Add the margarine by the tablespoonful, cutting it into the flour with your fingers or a pastry cutter, until the flour appears pebbly.

2. Mix together 4 tablespoons of the ice water with the apple cider vinegar. Drizzle in 2 tablespoons of the water/vinegar mixture and knead the dough, adding more water until it holds together. You may need only the 3 tablespoons, but add up to 2 more tablespoons if needed.

3. Divide the dough in two, press into two disks, and refrigerate until ready to use, or use as directed in the recipe.

Slices

Buckwheat flour is very delicate, so be a little more gentle when working with this crust.

PRESS-IN ALMOND CRUST

MAKES ONE 9-INCH PIE CRUST OR ONE 9- OR 10-INCH TART PAN CRUST

GIVE YOUR ROLLING PIN a time out with this nutty crust that's pressed directly into the pie or tart pan. The gluten-free variation produces a delicate, crumbly crust that's great with PEAR FRANGIPANE TART (page 139).

⅔ cup sliced almonds

1 cup all-purpose flour

2 tablespoons sugar

½ teaspoon salt

4 tablespoons canola oil

3 or more tablespoons cold almond
milk

1. Pour the almonds into a food processor and pulse into a fine meal, then add the flour, sugar and salt and pulse to combine. Continue to pulse and stream in canola oil, then pulse in 3 tablespoons of the almond milk. The mixture should hold together when pressed between your fingertips; if it still feels too crumbly mix in one additional tablespoon of almond milk at a time.

2. Lightly spray a tart pan with nonstick cooking spray and sprinkle in the crust mixture. Press it into the bottom and sides of the pan.

Variation

GLUTEN-FREE ALMOND CRUST: Substitute ⅔ cup certified gluten-free oat flour plus ⅓ cup rice flour for the all-purpose flour.

FRUIT PIES

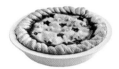

WHEN WE CLOSE our eyes and dream of pie, fruit is usually what we see. Tangy cherry pie paired with a cup of black coffee at the diner, our first taste of spring in the form of a tart and sweet strawberry rhubarb crumb, blueberry pie at the center of attention in a July picnic spread. Fruit pies are usually our first loves and often the easiest pie to master with a few tricks and tips. Nothing beats those telltale, luscious streaks of color staining a white plate, letting the world know "I just had pie, and man, it was good."

Psst . . . looking for apple and other autumnal desserts? This chapter mostly covers spring and summer fruit. Head on over to the Harvest chapter for all your apple-y needs.

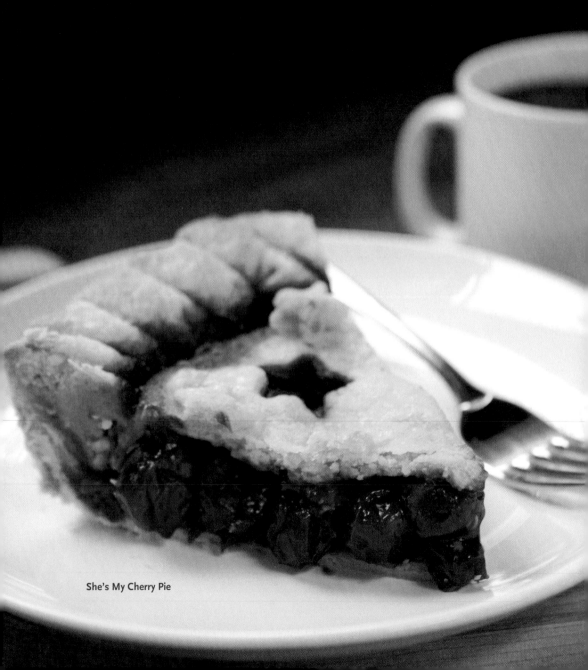

She's My Cherry Pie

SHE'S MY CHERRY PIE

PURE, SIMPLE PERFECTION—this is the cherry pie that makes everyone fall in love with you. Definitely do either a lattice top or a cutout crust to ensure that it's love at first sight!

1 recipe **BUTTERY DOUBLE CRUST** (page 37), rolled out and fit into a 9-inch pie plate

FILLING:

5 cups pitted tart cherries

¾ cup sugar

¼ cup cornstarch

⅛ teaspoon salt

TOP CRUST:

Nondairy milk for brushing

2 tablespoons sugar

1. Preheat the oven to 425°F. In a large mixing bowl, mix together all of the filling ingredients and set aside.

2. Add the filling to the prepared pie shell. Cover it with the top crust, pinch the edges together, trim the excess dough to about an inch, and crimp.

3. Brush the top of the pie with nondairy milk and sprinkle on sugar. Bake for 20 minutes, lower the heat to 350°F, and bake for another 30 minutes. The crust should be golden and the filling should be bubbly. Place pie on a cooling rack and let cool for about half an hour before serving.

CHERRY PICKIN'

THIS RECIPE CALLS for tart or sour cherries, and only those will do. Sweet cherries are delicious on their own but baking them takes away their magic. So eat a bowlful of sweet cherries at a picnic, but leave the pie to the effervescent sour cherry.

The downside is that sour cherries are virtually impossible to find out of season and the season really only lasts for a handful of summer weeks. But that's okay; frozen sour cherries work magnificently and are already pitted to boot! When you are able to find them frozen, snatch them up, as they tend to go fast. And follow our frozen fruit tips on page 12 to make sure your pies are flawless.

If frozen sour cherries are absolutely impossible to find, your next best bet is jarred. The concern with jarred cherries is that they are stored in a sweetened syrup, so drain them before proceeding with this recipe and reduce the sugar by a tablespoon or two. But don't let the juice go to waste! Use it for a sweet cherry blast in lemonade or sangria.

☀ *Slices* ☀

A handheld cherry pitter is a good investment, especially one that will pit olives, too. You should be able to procure one for well under twenty dollars. Our advice is just to search Amazon for the one with the best reviews!

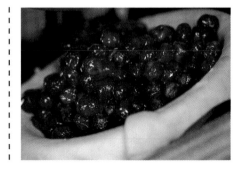

MAPLE-KISSED BLUEBERRY PIE

MAKES ONE 9-INCH PIE

A JUICY BLUEBERRY PIE with a hint of sweet maple, bright lemon, and a teeny bit of cinnamon. Using both maple syrup and maple extract adds super maple flavor goodness to an already perfect pie.

1 recipe double crust, either **BUTTERY** (page 37) or **OLIVE OIL** (page 39), rolled out and fit into a 9-inch pie plate

FILLING:

6 cups blueberries, fresh or frozen (see frozen fruit tips on page 12)

¼ cup pure maple syrup

⅓ cup sugar

1½ teaspoons maple extract

Grated zest of 1 lemon

2 teaspoons fresh lemon juice

½ teaspoon ground cinnamon

4 to 5 tablespoons cornstarch

Pinch of salt

TOPPING:

2 teaspoons sugar

1. Preheat the oven to 425°F. Combine all the filling ingredients in a large bowl, stirring with a rubber spatula until all the berries are coated.

2. Add the filling to the prepared pie shell. Cover with the top crust, pinch the edges together, trim the excess dough to about an inch, and crimp. Make five slits in the middle of the pie to let steam escape (a steak knife works great for this).

3. Sprinkle with the remaining 2 teaspoons of sugar. Bake the pie for 20 minutes, then lower the heat to 350°F and bake for another 30 minutes. The crust

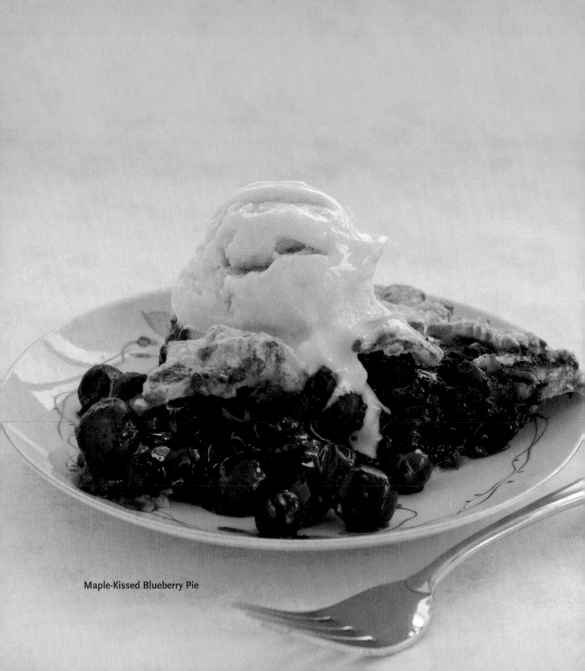

Maple-Kissed Blueberry Pie

should be golden and the filling should be bubbly. Place the pie on a cooling rack and let cool for about half an hour before serving.

Variation

BLUEBERRY THRILL PIE: Prefer your blueberries straight up? Omit maple syrup and extract and increase sugar to ½ cup.

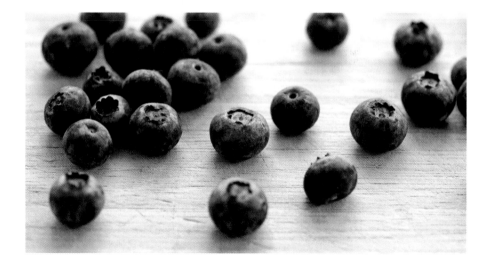

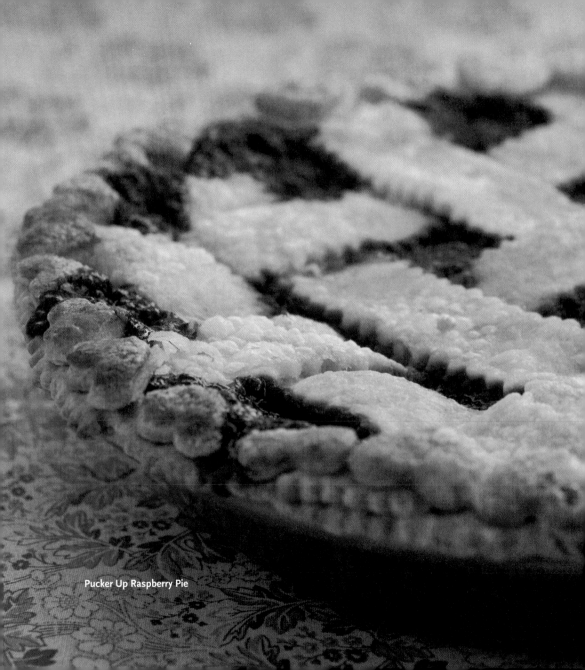
Pucker Up Raspberry Pie

PUCKER UP RASPBERRY PIE

THIS RASPBERRY PIE has a secret weapon . . . balsamic vinegar! Although you won't be able to detect it, it simply heightens the tart raspberry flavor like *whoa*. Even if you're using frozen berries they will taste like something special.

We always like to make a lattice top if there are red berries inside because how could you not? It would be crazy to hide all that vibrant color.

1 recipe BUTTERY DOUBLE CRUST (page 37), rolled out and fit into a 9-inch pie plate

FILLING:

5 cups raspberries, fresh or frozen (see tips on page 12)

3 tablespoons cornstarch

¾ cup sugar

2 tablespoons balsamic vinegar

⅛ teaspoon salt

1. Preheat the oven to 425°F.
2. In a large mixing bowl, mix together all of the filling ingredients and set aside.
3. Add the filling to the prepared pie shell. Create a lattice crust on top (see illustration on page 33), pinch the edges together, trim the excess dough to about an inch, and crimp.
4. Bake the pie for 25 minutes, then lower the heat to 350°F and bake for 30 to 35 more minutes. The filling should be bubbly and the crust lightly browned. Place pie on a cooling rack to let cool. It's very saucy at first, so give it an hour or so before slicing.

BLACKBERRY BRAMBLE PIE

THE EDGY, SULTRY SISTER of the raspberry lattice pie, this blackberry pastry is spiked with lots of lemon and a touch of blackberry liqueur. It's a flavorful, aromatic treat worth wading through the brambles for.

1 recipe **BUTTERY DOUBLE CRUST** (page 37), rolled out and fit into a 9-inch pie plate

FILLING:

6 generous cups blackberries, fresh or frozen (see tips on page 12)

Grated zest of 2 lemons

3 tablespoons fresh lemon juice

⅔ cup plus 1 tablespoon sugar

3 tablespoons blackberry liqueur or brandy

3 tablespoons cornstarch

¼ teaspoon ground cinnamon

1. Preheat the oven to 425°F. In a large mixing bowl, toss together the berries, lemon zest, lemon juice, ⅔ cup sugar, blackberry liqueur, cornstarch, and cinnamon.

2. Pile filling into pie crust and gently press down berries to even out the top. Assemble crust strips in a lattice design (see illustration on page 33) on top of pie and sprinkle with remaining 1 tablespoon of sugar.

3. Bake the pie for 20 minutes, then lower heat to 350°F and bake for another 30–35 minutes. The crust should be golden and the filling should be bubbly. Place pie on a cooling rack and let cool for about half an hour before serving.

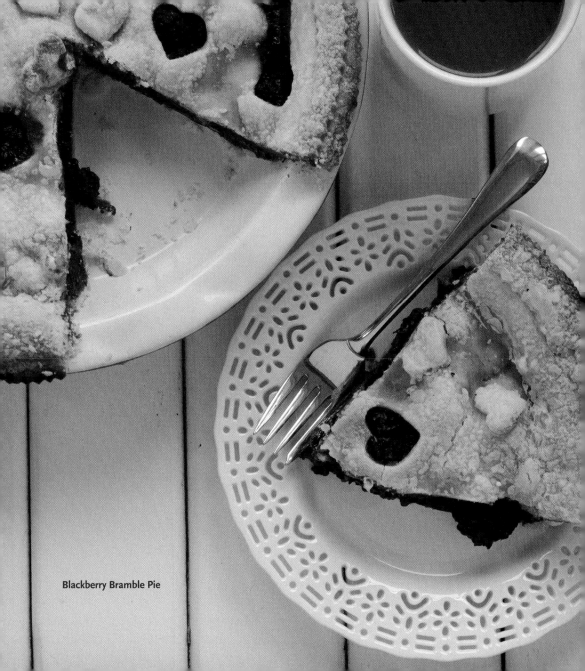

Blackberry Bramble Pie

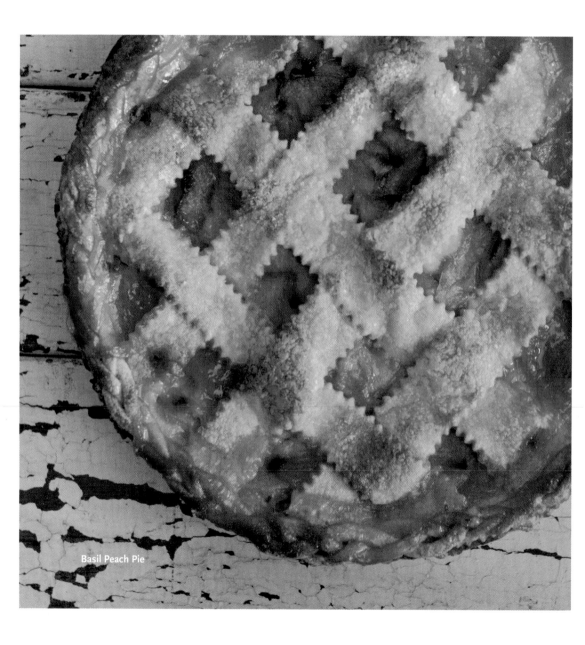

Basil Peach Pie

BASIL PEACH PIE

WE ARE VERY PARTICULAR about peach pie. It can be too brown-sugary, too almondy, too cinnamony, and just too obvious and unremarkable. This pie changes everything!

Using white sugar and a little lemon juice lets the peachy flavor shine. There are no spices, just honest peaches and one surprise ingredient (well, not a surprise to you because it's in the title) . . . fresh basil! It brings a springlike flair that's not at all in-your-face. We think if you took a bite without knowing what it was, you'd guess "enchanted faerie fruits" before basil. Try it on your friends and see!

1 recipe **BUTTERY DOUBLE CRUST** (page 37), rolled out and fit into a 9-inch pie plate

FILLING:

   6 cups sliced peaches (see tips)

   ¾ cup sugar

   ¼ cup all-purpose flour

   2 tablespoons fresh lemon juice

   8 average-size fresh basil leaves, snipped into small pieces

   ⅛ teaspoon salt

1. Preheat the oven to 425°F. Combine all the filling ingredients together in a large mixing bowl, then transfer them to the prepared pie shell.

2. Top the pie with the crust. Pinch the edges together, then trim the excess dough to about an inch and crimp the edges together.

3. Make five slits in the middle of the pie to let steam escape (a steak knife works great for this).

4. Bake for about 25 minutes. Lower the heat to 350°F and slip on the pie crust shield. Bake for an additional 30 minutes. Filling should

---

★ ★ ★

SCORE!

YOU NEED TO score and blanch the peaches to get the skins off. It's more fun than it sounds and will give you a great sense of accomplishment.

You'll need three things: (1) a big pot of boiling water; (2) a huge bowl for an ice bath; and (3) a slotted spoon to transfer the peaches.

To make the ice bath, fill the huge bowl with ice and cold water. Place it right next to the stove for fast transferring.

Now score the bottoms of the peaches by making an "X" in them with a knife. Place the peaches in the boiling water for one minute, and then transfer them to the ice bath using the slotted spoon. Let them cool for a few minutes, and then peel the skins off using the "X" you made at the bottom as the starting point.

Slice the peach in half, remove the pit, and cut into ¼-inch slices. Easy peasy, or eachy peachy!

---

be bubbling and the crust should be golden. Place the pie on a cooling rack and let cool for about half an hour before serving.

✴ Slices ✴

◆ For the best flavor, be super careful to use only the leaves of the basil and absolutely no stem. Also, make sure that the basil is as fresh and green as possible. Stems and dark spots can both cause bitterness, and you want only sweet peachiness.

◆ If using frozen peaches: You can totally use sliced frozen peaches here but the key to success is slicing them even more. Make sure that slices are around ¼ inch and ½ inch thick and definitely nowhere over ½ inch. Peaches should be partially thawed before adding them to the crust or it will affect the baking times. See frozen fruit tips on page 12.

STRAWBERRY RHUBARB CRUMB PIE

MAKES ONE 9-INCH PIE

WHOEVER FIRST THOUGHT that these two complete opposites would make a great pair should be given the biggest blue ribbon there is. Tart rhubarb and sweet strawberries, who can argue with that? A cinnamony crumb topping seals the deal (literally). Every pie is made better with vegan vanilla ice cream, but this one is especially so.

1 recipe SINGLE (AND LOVING IT!) PASTRY CRUST (page 42), rolled out and fit into a 9-inch pie plate, edges crimped

FILLING:

3 cups rhubarb, sliced ½ inch thick

4 cups strawberries, fresh or frozen (see tips page 12), sliced ¼ inch thick

⅔ cup sugar

2 tablespoons tapioca flour

2 tablespoons all-purpose flour

1 tablespoon fresh lemon juice

⅛ teaspoon salt

TOPPING:

1 cup all-purpose flour

⅓ cup brown sugar

2 tablespoons white sugar

¼ teaspoon salt

¼ teaspoon ground cinnamon

⅓ cup nonhydrogenated margarine, melted

1. Preheat the oven to 425°F. Combine all the filling ingredients together in a large mixing bowl.

2. In a separate bowl, combine flour, sugars, salt, and cinnamon for the topping. Drizzle in the margarine and use your fingers to swish around the mixture until crumbs form. Some of the topping is still

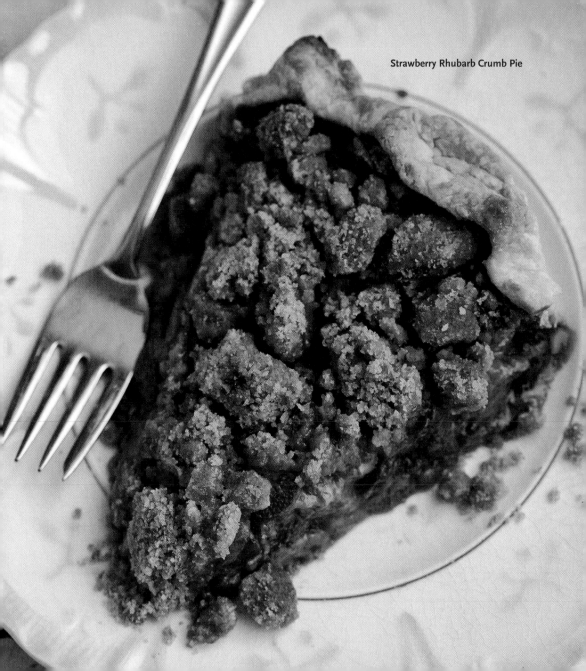

Strawberry Rhubarb Crumb Pie

going to be sandy and that's fine, just so long as you have mostly nice big crumbs.

3. Add the filling to the prepared pie shell and top with the crumb topping. Cover loosely with aluminum foil and poke a few holes in the foil to let steam escape.

4. Bake for about 20 minutes. Lower heat to 350°F and remove the foil. Bake for an additional 30 to 35 minutes. Filling should be bubbling and the crumb topping should be golden. Place on a cooling rack and let cool for about 30 minutes before serving.

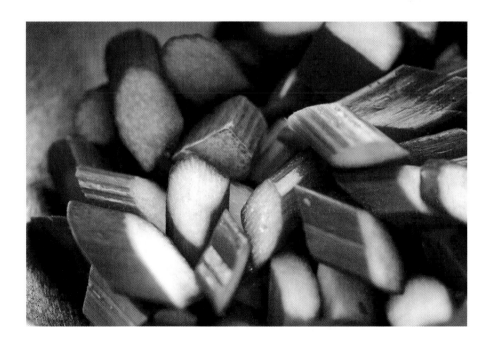

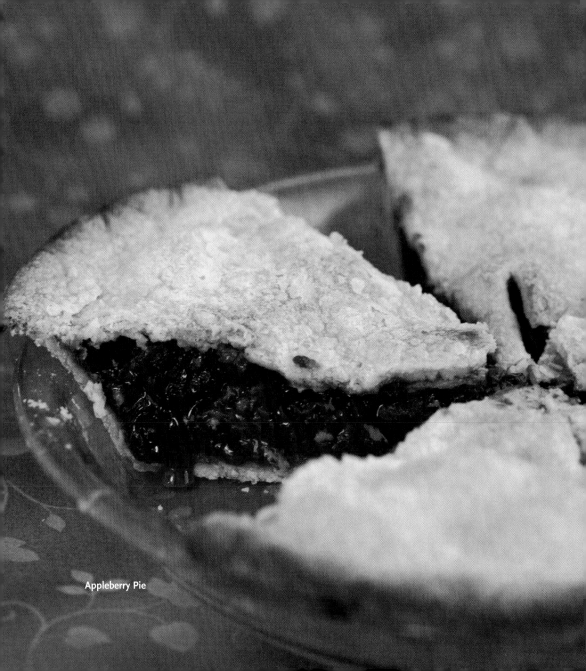

Appleberry Pie

APPLEBERRY PIE

NOT A MYSTERY FRUIT on its own, appleberry is the best of fruit pie worlds: the substantial, hearty texture of apples fused with sweet tart berries, be they fresh or frozen.

1 recipe **BUTTERY DOUBLE CRUST** (page 37) or **OLIVE OIL DOUBLE CRUST** (page 39), prepared and rolled as directed.

FILLING:

2 cups fresh blackberries, raspberries, blueberries, or a mix (about 10 ounces frozen berries)

4 cups peeled Granny Smith apples, sliced ¼ inch thick or less (about 1½ pounds)

2 tablespoons fresh lemon juice

⅔ cup sugar

¾ teaspoon ground cinnamon

Big pinch of ground nutmeg

4 tablespoons cornstarch

TOPPING:

2 tablespoons almond milk

1 tablespoon sugar

1. Preheat the oven to 425°F. Combine the filling ingredients in a large mixing bowl.

2. Fit the bottom crust into the pie plate, pile in the filling, and gently press down to get everything in. Cover with the top crust, pinch the edges together, trim excess dough to about an inch, and crimp. Make five slits in the middle of the pie to let steam escape (a steak knife works great for this).

3. Brush the top of the pie with almond milk and sprinkle with sugar.

4. Bake for 20 minutes. Reduce the heat to 350°F and continue baking 35 to 40 more minutes, or until the filling bubbles up through

the edges. Place the pie on a cooling rack and let cool for about 30 minutes before serving.

Variation

PEARBERRY PIE: Substitute a firm baking pear such as Bartlett or Bosc.

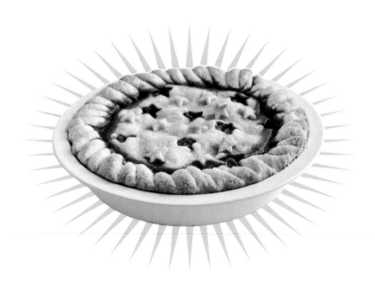

BLUEBERRY GINGER HAND PIES
with *Lemon Glaze*

HOW CAN PIE BECOME even more wonderful? Make it portable! Hand pies are the perfect treat to tuck into a lunchbox (your own or a child's). These are reminiscent of a toaster pastry with the soft dough and fruity center. This combo is a classic—sweet blueberries and spicy ginger heightened with a tart lemony glaze. And the ease of this hand pie (no finickiness, no dough scraps) makes them impossible to resist. Make some every week!

1 recipe **PUFFY PIE DOUGH** (page 41)

FILLING:

1 pound blueberries, fresh or frozen (see tips page 12)

⅓ cup sugar

1 tablespoon cornstarch

1 tablespoon tapioca powder

1 tablespoon fresh lemon juice

1 tablespoon finely grated fresh ginger

1 teaspoon pure vanilla extract

GLAZE:

3 tablespoons fresh lemon juice (plus more if needed)

1 cup confectioner's sugar, sifted

1 teaspoon finely grated lemon zest

¼ teaspoon pure vanilla extract

1. Divide the prepared dough into two logs about 6 inches long, wrap with plastic wrap, and chill for 30 to 45 minutes.
2. Combine all filling ingredients together in a mixing bowl.
3. Preheat the oven to 400°F and line two large, rimmed baking sheets with parchment paper.

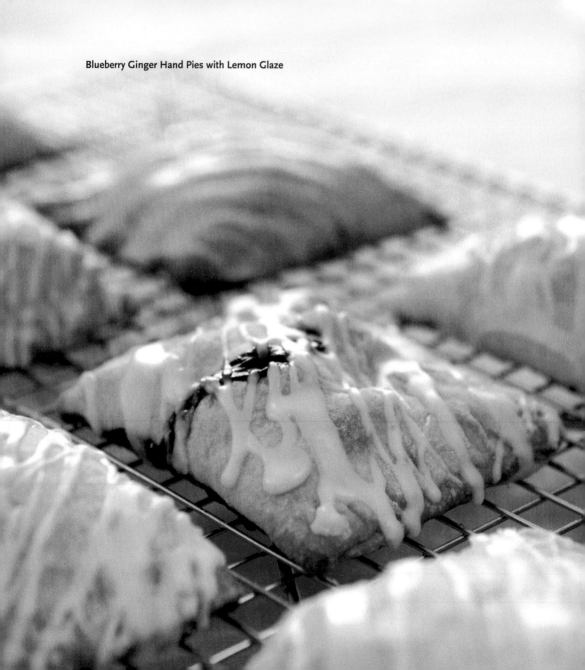

Blueberry Ginger Hand Pies with Lemon Glaze

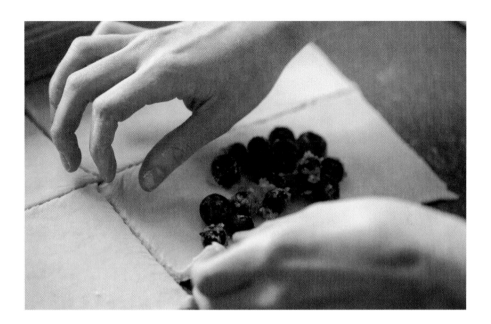

4. On a lightly floured surface, roll a dough log into a roughly 14 × 7-inch rectangle. Trim the edges with a paring knife so that they're even.

5. Slice the rectangle in half to form two squares. Slice the squares in half so that you have four smaller rectangles.

6. To form the hand pie: Dip your fingertips in water and use them to wet the edges of a pastry rec-tangle. Scoop a scant ¼ cupful of filling into one half of the pastry and fold it over, quickly running your finger along the edges to press them closed. Now press a fork into the pastry edges to create a pretty crimped pattern and to seal them well. If a little juice drips out, that's okay.

7. Transfer the hand pie to a baking sheet and continue with the oth-ers. When all four pies are formed, continue making pies with the other log of dough and place those on a separate baking sheet.

8. Create three slits in each hand pie to let steam escape.

9. Bake for 30 to 35 minutes on two separate racks, switching the pans between racks halfway through baking so that they bake evenly. The pies are ready when the edges are lightly browned and the filling is bubbly. Remove from oven and let cool for 5 minutes. Remove pies from the trays and let cool completely. (You can just lift the parchment to move the pies to a different surface.)

10. When pies are still a little bit warm, prepare the glaze by vigorously mixing the ingredients together. The consistency should be pretty drippy but not watery. If the glaze seems too stiff, add a

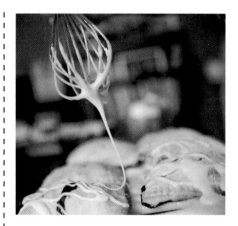

smidge more lemon juice. Use a spoon or whisk to drizzle glaze over the pies in a splattery pattern. To prevent a big mess, just place your cooling rack right over the sink to catch the excess glaze.

11. Continue to let the pies cool. If the glaze still seems sticky, place the pies in the freezer for 5 minutes to make it set.

STRAWBERRY FIELD HAND PIES

MAKES EIGHT HAND PIES

THERE'S SOMETHING SO DARLING about sticky strawberry juice creeping out of the edges of a hand pie. The dough is a little puffy with a nice crunchy bite on top from sugar, while the tangy sweet (but not too sweet!) juice oozes onto your tongue. It's so summery it'll make you want to don a sundress and go strolling through a field. But don't do that if it's winter. These would make a great addition to brunch.

1 recipe **PUFFY PIE DOUGH** (page 41)

FILLING:

1 pound frozen strawberries

¼ cup sugar, plus extra for sprinkling

2 tablespoons cornstarch

1 tablespoon fresh lemon juice

1 teaspoon pure vanilla extract

1. Divide the prepared dough into two logs about 6 inches long, wrap with plastic wrap, and chill for 30 to 45 minutes.

2. Let the frozen strawberries thaw just to the point where they are easy to slice.

3. Preheat the oven to 400°F and line two large, rimmed baking sheets with parchment paper.

4. To prepare the filling, slice strawberries into ¼-inch slices. Put them in a mixing bowl and mix with ¼ cup sugar, cornstarch, lemon juice, and vanilla extract. Place the filling in the freezer while you roll out the dough.

5. On a lightly floured surface, roll a dough log into a roughly 14 × 7-inch rectangle. Trim the edges with a paring knife so that they're even.

6. Slice the rectangle in half to form

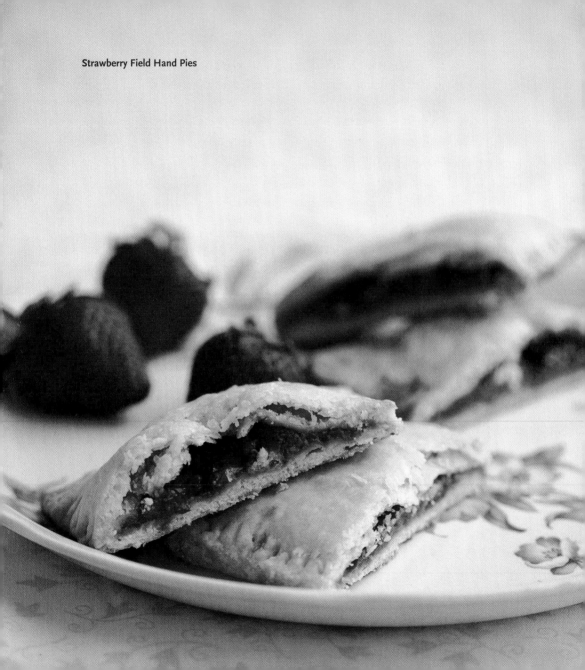

Strawberry Field Hand Pies

two squares. Slice the squares in half so that you have four smaller rectangles.

7. Remove the filling from the freezer. Have a cup of water at the ready. To form the hand pie, dip your fingertips in water and use them to wet the edges of a pastry rectangle. Scoop a scant ¼ cupful into one half of the pastry and fold it over, quickly running your finger along the edges to press it closed. Now press a fork into the edges to create a pretty crimped pattern and to seal them well. If a little juice drips out, that's okay.

8. Transfer the hand pie to a baking sheet and continue with the others. When all four pies are formed, continue making pies with the other log of dough and place those on a separate baking sheet.

9. Brush water on top of each pastry and sprinkle with a little sugar.

Create three slits in the dough to let steam escape.

10. Bake for 30 to 35 minutes on two separate racks, switching the pans between racks halfway through baking so that they bake evenly. The pies are ready when the edges are lightly browned and the filling is bubbly. Remove from oven and let cool for 5 minutes. Remove pies from the trays and let cool completely. (You can just lift the parchment to move the pies to a different surface.) Now eat in a sundress.

✳ *Slices* ✳

The secret to using strawberries in pastry is "work quick and work cold." Frozen strawberries are perfect here because the juice won't be too juicy and unruly while you're prepping. Even if you're using fresh strawberries, freeze them first. It will make them much easier to work with, because you want that juice creeping out of the dough, not splattered all over the place.

STRAWBERRIES & CREAM TARTS

MAKES SIX 4-INCH TARTS

IF SIMPLE AND PRECIOUS is how you like your desserts, then these are the tarts for you. Buttery shortbread and ambrosial strawberries are topped off with a luscious, melt-in-your mouth cream. These would be perfect for a tea party or gossipfest.

1 recipe **SHORTBREAD TART SHELL** (page 44)

1 recipe **SWEET COCONUT CREAM** (page 201)

FILLING:

4 cups strawberries, sliced ¼ inch thick (about 1½ pounds)

2 tablespoons cornstarch

2 tablespoons fresh lemon juice

⅓ cup sugar

PREPARE THE TARTS:

1. Distribute handfuls of shortbread crust equally among the tart pans. One by one, firmly press the dough into the sides and bottom of the tart pan.

2. Now poke the shells all over with a fork and place in the freezer for about 30 minutes. This part is important because the freezing and the poking will prevent the crust from puffing up when you par-bake.

1. Preheat the oven to 375°F. Remove the tarts from the freezer and place on a large, rimmed baking sheet. Bake for 10 minutes. Remove them from the oven and set aside (but keep the oven turned on to bake the tarts in a bit).

2. While the crust is baking, mix together all the filling ingredients.

The strawberries will release some juice, which will provide the sauce for the tarts.

3. When the tart pans are cool enough to handle a bit, line the strawberries around the circumference of the crust in an overlapping layer. Don't use the end pieces to line; instead pile them cut side down in the center of the tart.

4. Assemble all the tarts, and then spoon some of the juice over all the strawberries. It's okay if there are some strawberries left over; it is better to have some left over than to overfill the tarts.

5. Bake for 25 to 30 minutes, until the crust is lightly browned and the filling is bubbly. Remove from the oven and let cool until they are easy to handle (but still a bit warm.)

6. Now spoon some Sweet Coconut Cream over each tart, while they are still warm, so that it gets a bit melty. Serve warm, or, equally yummy, wait till the cream melts a bit and then chills, so that the strawberries are peeking out of the cream.

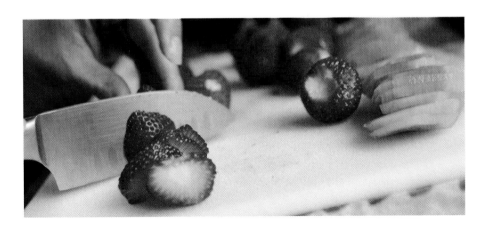

GINGER PEACH PANDOWDY

PANDOWDY ISN'T DOWDY AT ALL! It's a charming, old-timey treat, something like a single-crust fruit pie flipped upside down but easier to make than traditional pie. A simple concept, too, if you're not the type for fussy pie decorating: Fill a deep-dish pie plate with fruity goodness, top with a pastry crust, and halfway through baking, slice the top into pieces and smash down. When done baking you'll have a delectable mash of crisp crust drenched in sticky fruit juices on top with lush moist dough and fruit underneath. We love this playful dessert; it's great for use with repurposed frozen crusts (see page 11) that might not be so pretty after thawing but get a delicious new lease on life as a pandowdy!

1 recipe **SINGLE (AND LOVING IT!) PASTRY CRUST** (page 42) or thawed frozen crust

FILLING:

2 pounds peaches, pitted and skins removed (see tips for **BASIL PEACH PIE**, page 66)

⅔ cup sugar

3 tablespoons cornstarch

3 tablespoons finely minced candied ginger

2 teaspoons lemon juice

¼ teaspoon ground nutmeg

1. Preheat the oven to 425°F and have ready a ungreased, ceramic deep-dish 10-inch pie plate. Roll out crust to a 12-inch circle and keep chilled until ready to use.

2. Slice peaches into ½-inch pieces and pour into the pie plate. Sprinkle with remaining filling ingredients and toss to completely coat slices, then slide or roll crust on top. Gently press crust onto filling and bake for 20 minutes. Reduce the oven heat to 350°F.

3. Remove the pie from the oven and with a thin, sharp knife slice crust into diamonds about 1 inch wide, then use the back of a wide spoon to mash down the crust diamonds into the filling; some of the juices should seep over the crust. Return the pie to the oven and bake another 35 to 40 minutes or until the top is golden and the fruit is actively bubbling through the crust. Move the pie to a cooling rack for 20 minutes, then spoon warm pandowdy into serving bowls, top with a favorite vegan ice cream, and serve it up!

Variation

PLUMMY PANDOWDY: Substitute peak summer red and black plums for peaches. Peeling is optional. Or try a mix of plums, peaches, and apricots!

BLUEBERRY-LEMON CORN BISCUIT COBBLER

MAKES 6 TO 8 SERVINGS

LEMONY CORN BISCUITS FLOAT BLISSFULLY in a sea of lemon-kissed blueberry goodness. Great made with frozen blueberries for a burst of summer cobbler flavor during that first snowfall.

BERRY MIXTURE:

- 5 cups frozen blueberries
- 2 tablespoons fresh lemon juice
- ⅓ cup sugar
- 4 teaspoons tapioca powder or cornstarch
- ½ teaspoon ground cinnamon

BISCUITS:

- ¾ cup unbleached flour
- ½ cup yellow cornmeal
- ¼ cup sugar
- 1½ teaspoons baking powder
- ¼ teaspoon baking soda
- Pinch of salt
- 4 tablespoons cold nonhydrogenated margarine
- 2 tablespoons soy milk

- 2 tablespoons lemon juice
- Grated zest of 1 lemon

TOPPING:

- 1 teaspoon sugar

1. Preheat the oven to 400°F. In a 10-inch, deep-dish ceramic pie plate, combine the frozen un-thawed berries, lemon juice, sugar, tapioca powder, and cinnamon. Transfer it to the oven and bake for 25 minutes, then remove the plate from the oven (but leave the oven on; you'll need it again.)

2. Ten minutes before the berries are removed from the oven, make the biscuit topping. In a large mix-

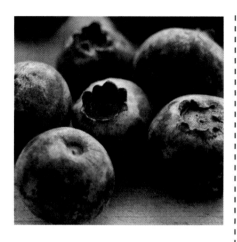

ing bowl, stir together the flour, cornmeal, sugar, baking powder, baking soda, and salt. Using a pastry cutter or your fingers, cut the margarine into the flour mixture until the mixture looks crumbly. In a measuring cup, stir together the soy milk and lemon juice and lemon zest, then sprinkle it over the dry ingredients and stir just enough to moisten ingredients to form a soft dough.

3. Gently gather the dough into a ball and on a lightly floured surface, pat it into a rectangle about 1 inch thick.

4. Use a sharp knife to slice the rectangle into eight squares, then arrange the dough squares on top of the hot blueberry mixture, spacing them evenly. Sprinkle the cobbler with 1 teaspoon of sugar.

5. Bake for another 20–22 minutes, until the biscuits are lightly browned and firm. Remove the cobbler from the oven, let it cool for 10 minutes, then serve warm with **RAD WHIP** (page 199) or any vegan vanilla ice cream.

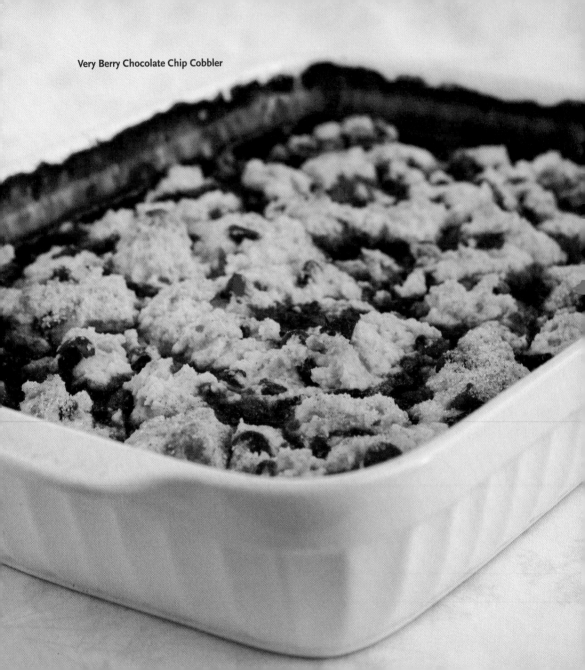

Very Berry Chocolate Chip Cobbler

VERY BERRY CHOCOLATE CHIP COBBLER

THIS IS A PLAYFUL COBBLER with lots of berry goodness and topped with chocolate chip–studded biscuits. It's perfect for a July 4th picnic or for one of those winter nights where the sun is nowhere in sight but you've got a few bags of mixed frozen berries. We love it with vegan vanilla ice cream.

FILLING:

10 cups berries (combo of blueberries, raspberries, and sliced strawberries; for frozen fruit, see tips on page 12)

2 tablespoons fresh lemon juice

1 cup sugar

2 tablespoons tapioca flour

¼ cup all-purpose flour

⅛ teaspoon salt

BISCUITS:

⅔ cup almond milk

1 tablespoon apple cider vinegar

2 cups all-purpose flour

2½ teaspoons baking powder

¼ teaspoon salt

¼ cup sugar

8 tablespoons nonhydrogenated margarine

1 cup chocolate chips

FOR SPRINKLING:

1 tablespoon sugar

½ teaspoon ground cinnamon

1. Prepare the filling: Preheat the oven to 425°F. Mix all the ingredients together in a 9 × 13-inch baking dish. Cover with aluminum foil and bake for 20 minutes.

2. In the meantime, prepare the biscuit topping. Combine the milk and vinegar in a measuring cup and set aside to curdle. In a large mixing bowl, sift together the flour, baking powder, and salt. Stir in sugar. Add the margarine by the tablespoonful, cutting it into the flour with your fingertips or a pastry cutter, until large crumbs form. Add the milk/vinegar mixture and gently stir a few times to combine. Fold in the chocolate chips.

3. On a separate plate, mix together the cinnamon and sugar. Remove the pan from the oven, discard the foil, and top the filling with tablespoon-size dollops of biscuit batter. Sprinkle with the cinnamon sugar.

4. Bake for an additional 20 minutes. The fruit should be very bubbly and the biscuits on top sunken in but firm where peeking out from the fruit.

5. Remove the cobbler from the oven and let cool for 15 minutes or so before digging in. Serve warm with vegan vanilla ice cream.

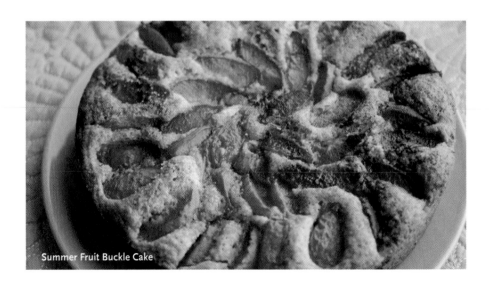

Summer Fruit Buckle Cake

SUMMER FRUIT BUCKLE CAKE

A BUCKLE IS AN OLD TIMEY DESSERT, an arrangement of fresh fruit atop cake batter; as the cake bakes, it rises and buckles around the roasting fruit for a rustic, hilly surface. Less juicy than a cobbler and closer to a coffee cake, this buckle stars the best fruit summer has to offer— apricots, peaches, plums and even berries—to wow brunch guests or partner up with an after- noon cup of coffee or tea.

¾ cup sliced almonds or ⅔ cup ground
    almonds
1½ cups all-purpose flour
2 teaspoons baking powder
½ teaspoon baking soda
½ teaspoon salt
¼ teaspoon ground cinnamon
¼ teaspoon ground cardamom
1 cup soy milk
2 teaspoons apple cider vinegar
⅔ cup sugar
⅓ cup canola oil
1½ teaspoons pure vanilla extract
½ teaspoon almond extract

TOPPING:

10 apricots or small ripe plums, 4 to 5
    medium-size peaches, or about 1
    pound fruit
1 tablespoon turbinado sugar
¼ teaspoon ground cinnamon

1. Preheat the oven to 350°F and line the bottom of a 9-inch round cake pan with a circle of parch- ment paper. Generously spray the bottom and sides of the pan with nonstick cooking spray.

2. In a blender or food processor pulse the sliced almonds into a fine meal (if not using almond meal). In a mixing bowl combine

the ground almonds with the flour, baking powder, baking soda, salt, cinnamon, and cardamom. In a large measuring cup stir together the soy milk and apple cider vinegar until mixture is curdled, then stir in the sugar, canola oil, vanilla extract, and almond extract.

3. Prepare the topping before stirring together the cake ingredients: Remove pits from apricots, plums, or peaches and cut fruit into ½ inch slices. Stir together the turbinado sugar and cinnamon.

4. Now create a well in the center of the dry cake mixture, pour in the soy milk mixture, and with a rubber spatula or wooden spoon stir just long enough to moisten all of the ingredients; a few small lumps are okay. Spread cake batter into the prepared pan and arrange the fruit in a spiral pattern on top of the cake; it's easiest to work from the outside edge toward the center. Sprinkle the top of cake with cinnamon sugar and bake on the

center rack of the oven for 45 to 55 minutes or until a toothpick inserted into the center of the cake comes out with a few moist crumbs (and not wet batter—the center of the cake should not be raw). Remove from the oven to a cooling rack; after 20 minutes place a dinner plate on top of the cake and flip the pan over. Peel off the parchment paper, place a serving plate on top of the cake and carefully flip it over one last time. Serve warm or at room temperature.

Variations

Substitute 2½ cups of washed, picked-over blueberries for orchard fruit. Stir 2 cups of the fruit into the cake batter before spreading in the pan, then sprinkle the remaining ½ cup over the top of the cake before baking. Or use a mix of pitted, sliced sweet cherries, raspberries, and blueberries.

For a peach melba buckle, sprinkle a handful of cleaned raspberries over sliced peaches!

CREAMY PIES

CHEESECAKES, PUDDING-FILLED PIES, and cream-filled tarts are now vegan dessert mainstays, too! We're in love with our litany of creamy dairy- and egg-free treats and are proud to present recipes that favor naturally vegan ingredients over faux dairy products. From the classic coconut cream pie to decadent peanut butter cheesecake to gorgeous fruit tarts, we've got your cravings for creamy confections covered.

CHOCOLATE GALAXY BANANA CHEESECAKE

MAKES ONE 9½-INCH CHEESECAKE

TOFU CHEESECAKE IS the new vegan classic with variations aplenty, all in search of that dense, creamy cheesecake experience. We love our version and can't wait to share it with the world: satisfying to prepare and baked just like a "real" cheesecake, with a mildly tart and creamy texture made possible without a drop of expensive, store-bought vegan cream cheese.

This cheesecake also freezes great, and double bonus, it tastes awesome partially thawed for a ridiculous semifreddo-like treat.

1 recipe GRAHAM CRACKER CRUST (page 46), or Chocolate Cookie Crust variation

FILLING:
½ cup whole unroasted cashews, soaked in water for 2 to 8 hours or until very soft
½ cup well-mashed banana (about 2 medium-size bananas)
1 (12–14 ounce) package silken tofu, drained
⅔ cup sugar
2 tablespoons coconut oil, room temperature
4 teaspoons cornstarch

1 tablespoon lemon juice
2 teaspoons pure vanilla extract
¼ teaspoon almond extract
¼ teaspoon sea salt
⅔ cup semisweet chocolate chips

1. Preheat the oven to 350°F. Lightly spray a 9-inch springform pan with cooking spray. Prepare the crust and press it very firmly into the pan. Bake for 10 minutes and move the pan to a cooling rack.

2. Meanwhile, prepare the filling: Drain the cashews and blend with the banana, tofu, sugar, coconut

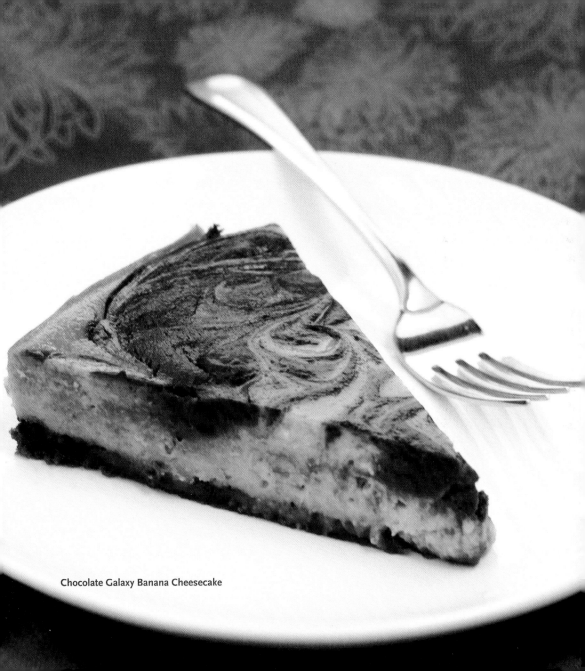

Chocolate Galaxy Banana Cheesecake

oil, cornstarch, lemon juice, vanilla and almond extracts, and sea salt. Blend until completely smooth and absolutely no bits of cashew remain.

3. Set aside ⅓ cup of batter and pour the rest into the crust. Melt the chocolate chips over a double boiler or in a glass bowl in the microwave. Stir the melted chips with a spatula until smooth; add reserved batter and stir until smooth.

4. Spoon dollops of chocolate batter randomly onto the cheesecake. Poke the end of a chopstick into a chocolate batter blob and gently swirl the top to create a marble-like pattern; repeat with the remaining chocolate blobs.

5. Bake the cheesecake for 50 to 55 minutes until the top is lightly puffed and the edges of the cake are golden.

6. Remove the cake from the oven and set on a cooling rack for 20 minutes, then move it to the fridge to complete cooling, at least 3 hours or even better, over-night. To serve, slice the cake with a thin, sharp knife dipped in cold water.

Variations

BANANA KAHLÚA CHEESECAKE: Stir ¼ cup of Kahlúa or other favorite coffee liqueur into the chocolate batter before swirling it into the cheesecake.

BANANA SPLIT CHEESECAKE: Serve each slice of cheesecake with a dollop of RAD WHIP (page 199), or use a pastry bag fitted with a large round nozzle for an elegant swirl. Lace it with chopped pineapple and CHOCOLATE DRIZZLE (page 203), sprinkle with chopped walnuts, and top with a cherry.

☀ Slices ☀

Cracks on the surface of your cheesecake got you down? To help prevent cracking, place another baking rack directly under the rack the cheesecake will bake on. On the bottom rack arrange another pie plate or similar oven-proof dish and fill with 2 cups of hot water just before baking the cheesecake. The added humidity will help prevent large cracks from forming.

BLUEBERRY BLISS CHEESECAKE

MAKES ONE 9½-INCH CHEESECAKE

BLUEBERRY CHEESECAKE WITH a syrupy blueberry topping. Total blueberry bliss! If you're using frozen blueberries, then a 12-ounce bag oughta do ya.

1 recipe cookie crust variation of the GRAHAM CRACKER CRUST (page 46), preferably Vanilla Cookie Crust

FILLING:
½ cup whole unroasted cashews, soaked in water for 2 to 8 hours or until very soft
1 cup blueberries
⅓ cup mashed banana (about 1 medium-size banana)
1 (12–14 ounce) package silken tofu, drained
¾ cup sugar
3 tablespoons coconut oil, room temperature
2 tablespoons cornstarch
½ teaspoon sea salt
¼ cup lemon juice
1 tablespoon pure vanilla extract

TOPPING:
¼ cup sugar
2 cups blueberries
1 tablespoon cornstarch
2 tablespoons lemon juice

1. Preheat the oven to 350°F. Lightly spray a 9-inch springform pan with cooking spray. Prepare the cookie crumb crust and press it very firmly into the pan. Bake for 10 minutes and move the pan to a cooling rack. Leave the oven on because you'll be baking the cheesecake in a little bit.

2. Meanwhile, prepare the filling: Drain the cashews and pour into a food processor or blender. Add the blueberries, banana, tofu, sugar, coconut oil, cornstarch,

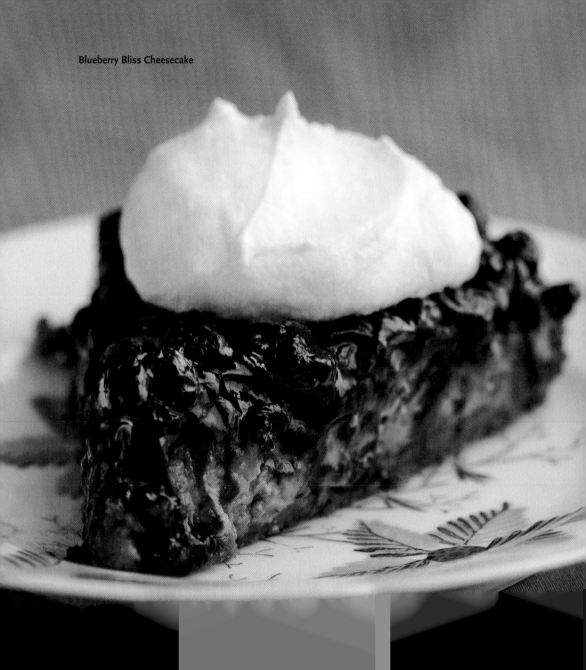
Blueberry Bliss Cheesecake

salt, lemon juice, and vanilla extract. Puree until very smooth; this could take up to 5 minutes depending on your blender. Pour the filling into the pan.

3. Bake the cheesecake for 55 to 60 minutes, until the top is lightly puffed and the edges of cake are pulling away from the pan. Remove it from the oven and let cool on a rack. In the meantime, prepare the topping.

4. Combine all the topping ingredients in a small saucepan. Stirring often, bring the mixture to a boil, so that the blueberries burst. Lower heat to a simmer and cook for about 5 more minutes. Remove the topping from the heat and pour it over the cheesecake.

5. Let the cake cool until it's okay to handle, about 30 minutes, and wrap it in plastic wrap. Place it in the fridge to set for about 2 hours.

6. Once completely set, release the springform and slice the cake with a sharp knife dipped in cold water.

RASPBERRY LIME RICKEY CHEESECAKE

MAKES ONE 9½-INCH CHEESECAKE

BAKING VEGAN CHEESECAKES can be habit-forming. Case in point, you may find yourself mysteriously compelled to whip up this tangy, lime- and raspberry-infused, soda fountain–inspired treat because it's amazing *and* you're maestro of vegan desserts. For the smoothest cheesecake, be sure to follow the instructions for preventing cracks on page 94.

1 recipe **GRAHAM CRACKER CRUST** (page 46)

FILLING:

½ cup whole unroasted cashews, soaked in water for 2 to 8 hours or until very soft

½ cup mashed banana (about 2 medium-size bananas)

1 (12–14 ounce) package silken tofu, drained

⅔ cup plus 1 tablespoon sugar

2 tablespoons coconut oil, room temperature

4 teaspoons cornstarch

4 tablespoons lime juice

Grated zest of 1 lime

2 teaspoons pure vanilla extract

¼ teaspoon almond extract

¼ teaspoon sea salt

RASPBERRY TOPPING:

1 (10-ounce) bag frozen raspberries, thawed at room temperature, juices retained

3 tablespoons sugar

½ teaspoon agar powder

½ teaspoon cornstarch

½ teaspoon lime juice

1. Preheat the oven to 350°F. Lightly spray a 9-inch springform pan with cooking spray. Prepare the crust and press it very firmly into the pan. Bake for 10 minutes and move the pan to a cooling rack.

Leave the oven on because you'll be baking the cheesecake in a little bit.

2. Meanwhile, prepare the filling: Drain the cashews and blend with mashed banana, tofu, sugar, coconut oil, cornstarch, lime juice, lime zest, vanilla and almond extracts, and sea salt. Blend until completely smooth and no bits of cashew remain. Pour the batter over the crust; tap the sides of the pan a few times to release any large air bubbles.

3. Bake the cheesecake for 45 to 50 minutes, until the top is lightly puffed and the edges of cake are golden. Remove it from the oven and let cool on a rack for 15 minutes. While the cake is cooling prepare the topping: In a small saucepan, combine the thawed raspberries, sugar, agar powder, cornstarch and lime juice. Bring the mixture to a simmer over medium heat and cook for 4 to 6 minutes, stirring occasionally, until thickened to the consistency of melted jam. Spoon the mixture onto the cake, working from the center and spreading it to the edges. Let the cake cool for 10 minutes, then move it to the fridge to complete cooling, at least 3 hours or even better, overnight. To serve, slice the cake with a thin, sharp knife dipped in cold water.

Variation

BLUEBERRY ORANGE CHEESECAKE: Use grated zest from one orange in place of lime and substitute orange juice for lime juice. Use blueberries in place of raspberries for the topping, replacing 2 tablespoons of lemon juice for the lime juice.

Slices

If you prefer a seedless raspberry topping, strain the berries after they have completely thawed but before cooking them. Use a fine mesh metal strainer and make sure to press out as much raspberry goo as possible.

KEY LIME PIE

THE TEXTURE RESEMBLES a creamy panna cotta, the flavor is pucker-your-lips tangy, and it will definitely satisfy the lime lover in your life. Remember to zest your limes before squeezing out the juice. if you can find Key Limes, then great! But it tastes wonderful with regular old limes, as well.

1 recipe GRAHAM CRACKER CRUST (page 46), parbaked for 10 minutes at 350°F

FILLING:

- 1½ cups unsweetened almond milk
- 2 tablespoons tapioca flour
- 2 teaspoons agar powder
- 1 (16 ounce) can coconut milk at room temperature
- ½ cup sugar
- ⅔ cup fresh lime juice
- 1 tablespoon finely grated lime zest
- 1 teaspoon pure vanilla extract

1. In a saucepot, mix together almond milk, tapioca flour, and agar powder. Turn heat up to a boil and stir constantly for about 5 minutes, until slightly thickened.

2. Very slowly whisk in the coconut milk. Then add sugar, lime juice, and zest. Whisk often for about 10 minutes, then turn off heat and add vanilla extract.

3. Pour into pie shell and let cool on the counter for about half an hour, just so that it isn't steaming like mad. Refrigerate for at least 3 hours, until fully set. Garnish with lime slices and RAD WHIP (page 199).

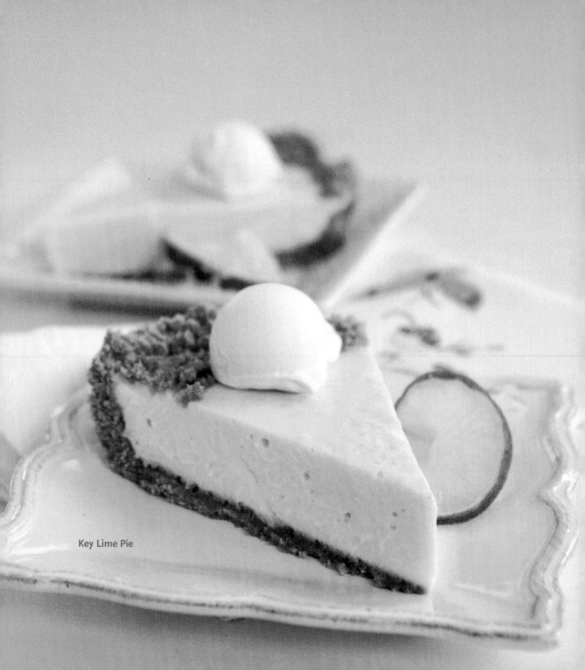

Key Lime Pie

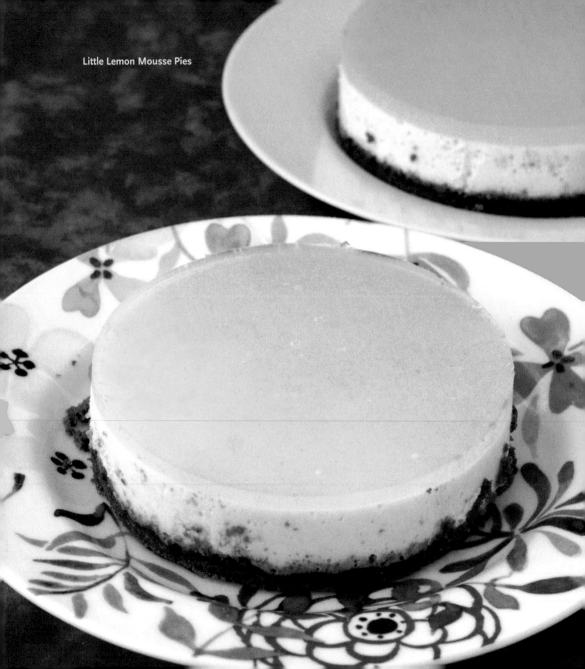

Little Lemon Mousse Pies

LITTLE LEMON MOUSSE PIES

MAKES FOUR 4-INCH PIES

A SUPER LIGHT AND CREAMY lemon mousse veiled with a glossy topping that is even lemonier. These little pies are truly a sight to behold. They're like an upside down lemon meringue pie! The gingersnap crust is a perfect complement.

This recipe makes four pies but you might want to split them between two people. It also works as a 9-inch pie in a springform pan.

1 recipe **GINGERSNAP CRUST** (page 48)

FILLING:

½ cup whole unroasted cashews, soaked in water for 2 to 8 hours or until very soft

1 (13-ounce) can coconut milk at room temperature

½ cup plain unsweetened almond milk or nondairy milk of your choice

½ teaspoon agar powder

⅔ cup sugar

3 tablespoons coconut oil

½ cup fresh lemon juice

2 tablespoons lemon zest

2 teaspoons pure vanilla extract

TOPPING:

¾ cup water

1 tablespoon cornstarch

⅓ cup fresh lemon juice

⅓ cup sugar

¾ teaspoon agar powder

¹⁄₁₆ teaspoon turmeric

2 teaspoons finely grated lemon zest

1. Preheat the oven to 350°F. Divide the crust between 4 four-inch springform pans, pressing it firmly into each pan. Bake for 10 minutes at 350°F, then remove them from the oven and let cool.

2. Drain the cashews and place them

in a food processor or blender. Blend them with the coconut milk until totally smooth, scraping down the sides of the bowl occasionally. This can take up to 5 minutes depending on the strength of your machine.

3. In the meantime, stir together the almond milk, agar powder, and sugar in a small (2-quart) saucepot.

4. Bring the mixture to a boil, stirring pretty consistently. Once boiling, lower the heat so that you're just getting small bubbles. Let cook for about 5 minutes, then add the coconut oil and mix until melted.

5. With the food processor running, stream the hot mixture in until thoroughly blended, then add the lemon juice, lemon zest, and vanilla extract and pulse a few times to combine.

6. Transfer the mixture to the prepared pie crust and refrigerate until set, about 4 hours. The filling is very thin at first, but that is how it's supposed to be.

7. When pie is just about set, prepare the topping: Stir together all the ingredients in a small saucepot. Bring the mixture to a boil, then lower the heat and cook for about 5 minutes. Pour the topping over the pies and place them back in the fridge to set for another hour.

8. When everything is set, undo the springform pans and serve!

LUXURY PISTACHIO PUDDING PIE

MAKES ONE 9-INCH PIE

WHEN ONLY THE FINEST WILL DO for the pistachio pudding fanatic in your life: a velvety pudding pie with true pistachio flavor, crowned by a ring of gleaming candied nuts. Artificially flavored pudding mixes need not apply when there is sweetened pistachio paste in this world. Love'n Bake makes a gorgeously green, decadent, and reasonably priced paste (look online for the best deals)—one can will set you up for two pies and it lasts forever when kept tightly sealed in the fridge. Or look for more expensive, gourmet organic pistachio pastes from Italy if you're a high-rolling pie gourmet—or make your own (see instructions that follow).

1 prepared, baked pie crust, either a cookie crust variation of the GRAHAM CRACKER CRUST (page 46), or SINGLE (AND LOVING IT!) PASTRY CRUST (page 42)

TOPPING:

¼ cup shelled pistachios

3 tablespoons sugar

2 tablespoons water

Pinch of salt

PUDDING:

⅓ cup plus 1 tablespoon sweetened pistachio paste

1¼ cups coconut milk

¼ cup sugar

1¼ teaspoons pure vanilla extract

⅛ teaspoon almond extract

Pinch of salt

1¼ cups unsweetened plain almond milk

¾ teaspoon agar powder

3 tablespoons cornstarch

1. Make the topping first. In a small skillet, combine the pistachios, sugar, and water. Bring the mixture to a simmer, stirring occasionally with a wooden spoon or heatproof rubber spatula. The

mixture will bubble, the water will evaporate, and the nuts will become encrusted with sugar; this should take about 10 to 12 minutes, so take your time. Continue to cook the nuts; the sugar will then begin to turn golden and melt somewhat, creating a light golden brown glaze. When the nuts look slightly syrupy, sprinkle them with salt and transfer them to a lightly oiled baking sheet or silicon mat. Separate any clumps and when cool, use a chef's knife to coarsely chop the nuts.

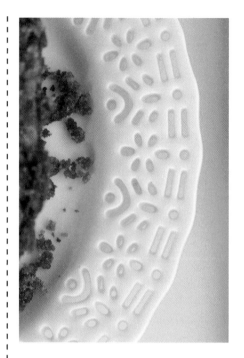

2. To make the pudding, in a blender pulse together the pistachio paste, coconut milk, sugar, vanilla extract, almond extract, and salt. Separately, in a small saucepan, pour ¾ cup of the almond milk and sprinkle it with the agar powder. Bring the milk to a simmer and cook over medium heat, stirring occasionally, for 6 minutes. In a measuring cup, whisk together the remaining ½ cup almond milk and the cornstarch, then slowly pour it into the simmering milk mixture and cook until thickened, about 3 to 4 minutes. Quickly scrape this into the blender with the pistachio mixture and pulse until creamy.

3. Pour the pudding into the prepared baked crust. Gently tap the sides of the pie to release any

large air bubbles. Let stand for 10 minutes, then sprinkle the candied pistachios around the edges of the pie. Transfer the pie to the refrigerator to cool completely, at least 3 hours, and carefully slice with a sharp knife dipped in cool water.

HOMEMADE PISTACHIO PASTE

1. In a food processor, pulse 1 cup of shelled, unsalted green pistachios and 1 tablespoon grapeseed oil or almond oil. Pulse until the nuts are as creamy and smooth as you can make them, scraping the sides of the processor frequently. Then pulse in 2 to 3 tablespoons of confectioner's sugar until a creamy paste is achieved.

Slices

The oil will separate in the can of pistachio paste, so open it carefully to avoid spilling oil everywhere. To blend the oils back into the paste, dump the entire contents of the can into a mixing bowl and use a rubber spatula to cream together. Store unused paste in a small, tightly covered container in the refrigerator.

COCONUT CREAM PIE

SINK YOUR FORK into a creamy cloud of heaven! This is pure coconut decadence. Just try to keep from sneaking into this in the middle of the night.

1 recipe **GRAHAM CRACKER CRUST** (page 46), Vanilla Cookie Crust variation

FILLING:

- ½ cup whole unroasted cashews, soaked in water for 2 to 8 hours or until very soft
- 1 (13-ounce) can coconut milk, at room temperature
- ¾ cup plain unsweetened almond milk or nondairy milk of your choice
- ½ teaspoon agar powder
- ⅔ cup sugar
- 3 tablespoons coconut oil
- 1 teaspoon pure vanilla extract
- 1 teaspoon coconut extract or an additional teaspoon of vanilla
- 1½ cups shredded coconut

MAKE IT FANCY:

Top each slice with **RAD WHIP** (page 199) and sprinkle with flaked coconut.

1. Preheat the oven to 350°F. Par-bake the crust for 10 minutes, then remove it from the oven and set aside.
2. Drain the cashews and place them in a food processor or blender. Blend them with the coconut milk until totally smooth, scraping down the sides occasionally. This can take up to 5 minutes depending on the strength of your machine.
3. In the meantime, stir together the almond milk, agar powder, and

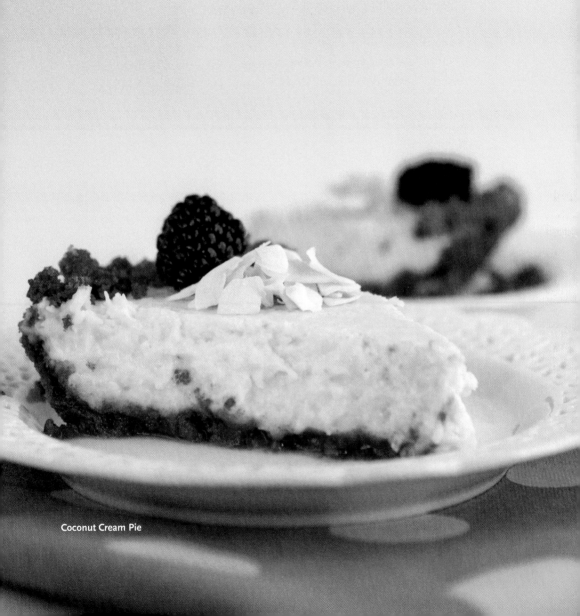
Coconut Cream Pie

sugar in a small (2-quart) sauce-pot.

4. Bring the mixture to a boil, stirring pretty consistently. Once boiling, lower the heat so that you're just getting small bubbles. Let cook for about 5 minutes, then add the coconut oil and mix until melted.

5. With the food processor running, stream the hot mixture in until thoroughly blended, then add the extracts and pulse a few times to combine. Stir in the shredded coconut, but don't blend it again, just mix it with a spatula—you want the coconut to remain intact.

6. Transfer the mixture to the prepared pie crust (being careful not to overfill) and refrigerate until set, 3 to 5 hours. The filling is very thin at first, but that is how it's supposed to be, so don't worry; it will thicken as it sets. Once set, slice and serve!

Variation

COCONUT LIME CREAM PIE: For ¼ cup of the almond milk, substitute ¼ cup fresh lime juice. Along with the shredded coconut, add 2 teaspoons lime zest and mix.

Slices

There may be a little leftover filling, so just pour it into a cup and let it set. Now you'll have a creamy taste for yourself without having to destroy the pie.

STRAWBERRY KIWI CRÈME TART

MAKES ONE 9½- TO 10-INCH TART

IN THE LAND of beautiful pastries, nothing gets wistful looks or noses pressed up against bakery windows like an elegant, French-inspired crème-filled tart topped with gleaming fresh fruit.

Well vegan dessert lover, the dream is now yours! Here's the tart that has it all: rich shortbread crust, luscious almond crème, and the sweet-tart pairing of strawberries and kiwis. The essential apricot jam topping keeps the fruit moist and adds a pretty shine. Enjoy making variations of this gorgeous tart with the best berries of the season: blueberries, strawberries, gooseberries, blackberries, and raspberries or even thinly sliced tropical fruits.

MAKE-AHEAD TIP: Prepare the tart shell up to a day in advance and store in a loosely covered container. The almonds can be toasted, cooled, and kept tightly covered until ready to use as well.

1 recipe **SHORTBREAD TART SHELL** (page 44), prepared in a 9½ or 10-inch tart pan, baked and cooled

FILLING:

1¼ cups plain unsweetened almond milk

½ teaspoon agar powder

2 tablespoons cornstarch

½ cup sugar

3 tablespoons coconut oil, room temperature

1 cup whole unroasted cashews, soaked in water for 2 to 8 hours or until very soft

1 teaspoon pure vanilla extract

½ teaspoon almond extract

¼ teaspoon lemon juice

Pinch of salt

½ pound strawberries, hulled and thinly sliced ¼ inch thick

½ pound kiwi fruit, peeled and thinly sliced ¼ inch thick

1 cup blackberries or blueberries

⅓ cup apricot jam, melted (see instructions below)

2 tablespoons sliced almonds, lightly toasted in a dry skillet over low heat

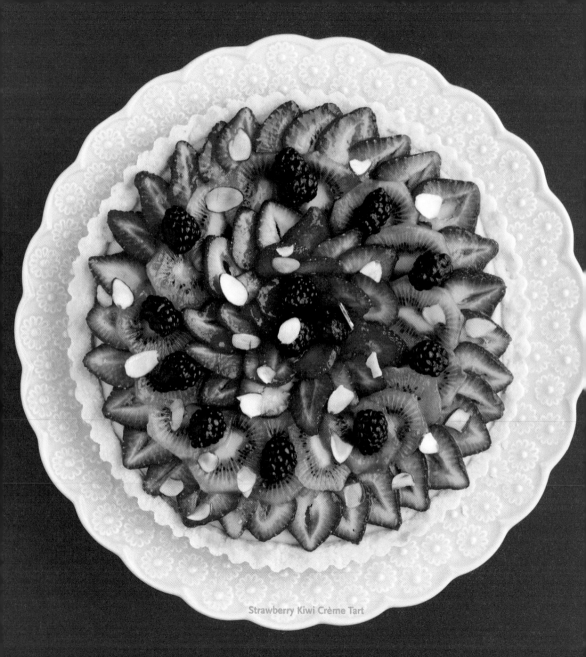

Strawberry Kiwi Crème Tart

1. In a large saucepan over medium-high heat, combine ½ cup of the almond milk with agar powder, bring it to a simmer, and cook for 6 minutes, stirring occasionally. In a measuring cup, whisk together the remaining almond milk and cornstarch, drizzle it into the almond milk and agar mixture, and cook for 4 to 5 minutes, stirring constantly with a wire whisk, until it thickens and no longer tastes starchy.

2. Now add the sugar and coconut oil and whisk until smooth, then right away pour it into the blender along with the drained cashews, vanilla extract, almond extract, lemon juice and salt. Blend until very smooth, about 2 to 3 minutes depending on your blender. Immediately pour the mixture into the prepared tart shell, filling it up to the top, and let stand at room temperature for 30 minutes.

3. Carefully arrange the sliced fruit in a spiral pattern on the crème, working from the outer edge toward the center, and when done dot the top with berries.

4. Melt the jam in a microwave-safe bowl by microwaving on high for 40 to 50 seconds (or in a small saucepan over medium heat), stirring occasionally until jam is loose, and use a pastry brush to gently brush the warm jam over the fruit. Make sure to cover all the sliced fruit with a thin layer of jam to prevent drying, then sprinkle the tart with toasted almonds and chill it. After at least 2 hours or when completely cool, slice with a sharp knife and serve immediately. This tart looks and tastes best if consumed the day it's made.

BANANA TOFFEE PUDDING PIE (BANOFFEE PIE)

MAKES ONE 9-INCH PIE

BANOFFEE PIE IS a British dessert with the best portmanteau name ever: bananas and toffee. This style of toffee more resembles a thick dulce de leche sauce (something we can always get down with), which goes on to encase a filling of bountiful fresh banana. Smother it all with Sweet Coconut Cream (or Rad Whip!) and chocolate shavings and it'll drive you bananas. Or banoffees.

SWEET COCONUT CREAM (page 201) made with less sugar to taste, or **RAD WHIP** (page 199)

1 SINGLE (AND LOVING IT!) PASTRY CRUST (page 42), baked and cooled

PUDDING:
> 1¼ cups coconut milk
> ⅔ cup dark brown sugar
> ⅓ cup plain unsweetened soy milk
> 3 tablespoons cornstarch
> ½ teaspoon pure vanilla extract
> 1 tablespoon nonhydrogenated margarine
> Pinch of salt
> 3 ripe bananas (about ¾ pound)

1-ounce piece semisweet chocolate bar, room temperature

1. Prepare the Sweet Coconut Cream or Rad Whip, cover tightly, and keep well chilled until ready to serve the pie.

2. In a small saucepan, combine the coconut milk and brown sugar over medium-high heat. Bring to a rolling boil, then reduce the heat to low. Simmer for 35 to 40 minutes, stirring occasionally, until the mixture is a deep caramel brown and slightly thickened.

3. In a measuring cup, whisk together the soy milk and cornstarch, then

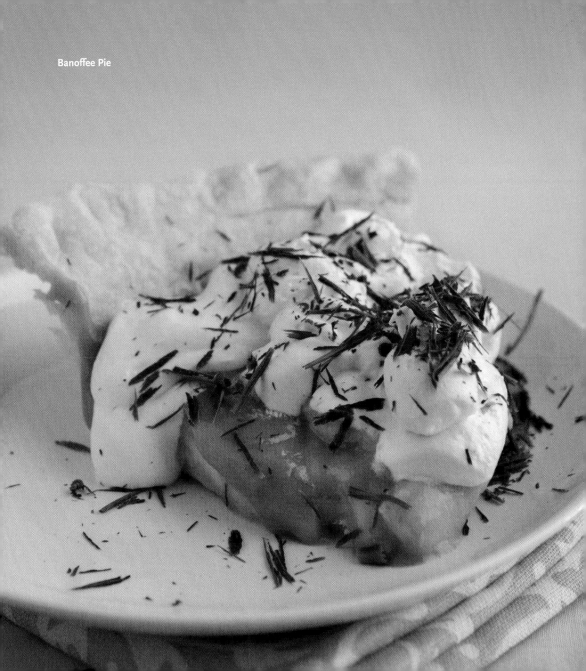

Banoffee Pie

pour it into the coconut milk mixture in a steady stream, whisking constantly. Continue stirring and cook until the mixture resembles a thick butterscotch pudding, about 4 to 5 minutes. Stir in the vanilla extract, margarine, and salt and remove the pudding from the heat.

4. Peel the bananas. Slice each banana in half crosswise and slice each half lengthwise into ¼-inch-thick pieces.

5. Spread a thin layer of pudding on the baked pie crust and place half the bananas on the pudding in an even layer. Cover the bananas with a thin layer of pudding, top with the remaining bananas, and cover with the remaining pudding. Use a rubber spatula to even out the top; make sure all of the bananas are encased in pudding to prevent excessive browning.

6. Gently wrap the top of the pie with plastic wrap, but don't let it touch the pudding. Move the pie to the refrigerator and chill for 2 hours or until completely cool.

7. Once the pie is cool, remove the plastic wrap and spoon the Sweet Coconut Cream or Rad Whip evenly over the top. Use a Y-shaped vegetable peeler to create the chocolate curls by running the blade on an angle along the chocolate bar, making as many chocolate curls as desired. For less mess do this directly over the pie. Serve immediately, or for a firmer pie let chill overnight. Use a sharp, thin knife dipped in cold water to slice up that banoffee.

Variation

COFFEE BANOFFEE PIE: Whisk 1 teaspoon instant coffee granules into the Sweet Coconut Cream or Rad Whip before spreading it over the pie. For a light-colored cream, use ½ to ¾ teaspoon of coffee extract instead of the granules.

✳ Slices ✳

The filling is very sweet and we recommend using half the amount of confectioner's sugar in the Sweet Coconut Cream. Rad Whip uses less sugar and it's unlikely you'll need to adjust anything.

CAPPUCCINO MOUSSE PIE

MAKES ONE 9-INCH PIE

FINALLY, A PIE FOR THE COFFEE LOVER. We love the texture of this pie! Lush and creamy, but still managing to be light and airy. There's a hint of chocolate in here, but only because it heightens the coffee flavor. Have a slice of this pie instead of your morning latte and you're all set.

1 recipe **GRAHAM CRACKER CRUST** (page 46), or Chocolate Cookie Crust variation

FILLING:
 ½ cup whole unroasted cashews, soaked in water for 2 to 8 hours or until very soft
 1 (16-ounce) can coconut milk at room temperature
 1 cup plain unsweetened almond milk or nondairy milk of your choice
 2 tablespoons instant coffee granules
 ½ teaspoon agar powder
 ⅔ cups sugar
 ¼ cup semisweet chocolate chips, melted
 1 teaspoon pure vanilla extract

OPTIONAL GARNISH:
 RAD WHIP (page 199) or store-bought vegan whipped topping
 ½ teaspoon ground cinnamon

1. Preheat the oven to 350°F and parbake the crust for 10 minutes, then remove from the oven and let cool.

2. Drain the cashews and place them in a food processor or Vita-Mix type thing. Blend them with the coconut milk until totally smooth, scraping down the sides occasionally. This can take up to 5 minutes depending on the strength of your machine.

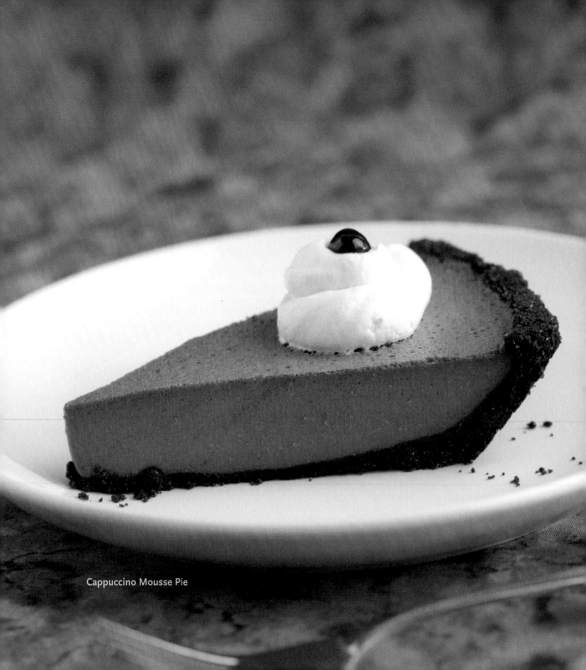

Cappuccino Mousse Pie

3. In the meantime, stir together the milk, coffee, agar powder, and sugar in a small (2-quart) saucepot.

4. Bring mixture to a boil, stirring pretty consistently. Once boiling, lower the heat so that you're just getting small bubbles. Let cook for about 5 minutes, then add the chocolate chips and mix until they're melted.

5. With the food processor running, stream the hot milk mixture in until thoroughly blended, then add the vanilla extract.

6. Transfer mixture to the prepared pie crust and refrigerate until set, 2 to 4 hours. Top with vegan whipped cream if desired and sprinkle with cinnamon.

CHAI-SPICED RICE PUDDING PIE

CREAMY RICE MAKES FOR A SURPRISING PIE with a really great texture. Aromatic jasmine rice is subtly flavored with chai tea bags, which would make it the perfect ending to an Indian-inspired dinner.

1 recipe GINGERSNAP CRUST (page 48), baked in a 350°F degree oven for 10 minutes

FILLING:
- 2¼ cups plain almond milk
- 1 (16-ounce) can coconut milk
- 1 cup uncooked jasmine basmati rice, rinsed
- ¾ cup sugar
- 1 teaspoon salt
- 4 chai tea bags
- 1 cinnamon stick
- 2 tablespoons cornstarch
- ¼ cup golden raisins (use brown raisins if you must; we just think golden are pretty)
- 2 teaspoons pure vanilla extract
- 2 tablespoons lemon juice

TOPPING:
- 2 teaspoons sugar
- ½ teaspoon ground cinnamon

1. Preheat the oven to 350°F.
2. Combine 1¾ cups of the almond milk, the coconut milk, rice, sugar, and salt in a small (2-quart) saucepan. Bring to a boil, then lower the heat. Add the tea bags and cinnamon stick and let simmer uncovered for about 30 minutes, or until the rice is mostly tender, stirring occasionally. Take care to stir gently and make sure that the mixture isn't wildly bubbling, or a tea bag may rip. If that does happen, it's not too big of a deal, just gently remove the bag.

3. When the rice is mostly tender, remove the tea bags and cinnamon stick. In a measuring cup, vigorously mix together the remaining ½ cup of almond milk and the cornstarch, until no big lumps remain. Stream the almond milk mixture into the rice pudding, stirring while you pour.

4. Mix in the raisins and cook for another 10 minutes, stirring occasionally. The rice should be very tender now, but if not, cook it for a few more minutes.

5. Turn off the heat and mix in the vanilla extract and lemon juice.

6. Pour the mixture into the prepared pie plate and let cool on the counter until it stops steaming. Wrap in plastic wrap and refrigerate for about 2 hours, or until fully set. Sprinkle with cinnamon sugar and serve.

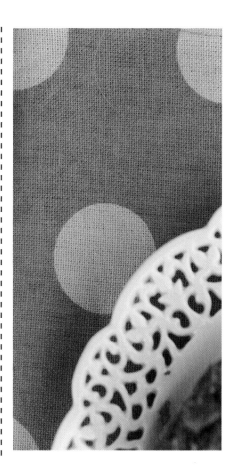

BANANA COOKIE CREAM PUDDING

BANANAS, VANILLA CREAM PUDDING, and vanilla cookie wafers have crept their way into the memories of countless dessert fans and into the pages of our pie book. Our version could be poured into a vanilla cookie pie crust (in place of using wafer cookies), or spooned artfully into parfait glasses, but we like to simply enjoy it "cobbler" style, in a rectangular dish or deep-dish pie plate. For additional homey charm line the edges of the dish with cookies resting on their edge to form a "crust"; for best results use larger round cookies and avoid using very small cookies that might float up into the pudding.

10 ounces vegan vanilla cookies such as Swedish vanilla snaps or wafers

3 large ripe bananas

1 (12–14 ounce) package silken tofu, drained

2 tablespoons coconut oil, room temperature

2½ teaspoons pure vanilla extract

¼ teaspoon almond extract

2 teaspoons lemon juice

⅛ teaspoon salt

Pinch of ground nutmeg

2 cups plain soy milk

½ teaspoon agar powder

2 tablespoons cornstarch

1 cup sugar

1. Remove 8–10 cookies from the package and with a food processor or rolling pin crush them into coarse crumbs. Set aside the remaining cookies and leave whole. Peel and slice the bananas on a diagonal into ½-inch slices.

2. Prepare the filling. In a blender, pulse together the tofu, coconut oil, vanilla extract, almond extract, lemon juice, salt, and nut-

meg until smooth. Then in a small saucepan combine 1 cup soy milk and the agar powder. Bring the mixture to a rolling boil over medium-high heat and cook for 30 seconds. Turn down heat to a simmer and cook, stirring occasionally, for 5 minutes.

3. Meanwhile, in a measuring cup whisk together the remaining 1 cup of soy milk and the cornstarch. Slowly pour it into the simmering soy milk mixture, then stir in the sugar and stir constantly until thickened, about 3 to 4 minutes.

4. Scrape this hot cooked mixture into the blender and pulse again until everything is smooth, scraping the sides of the blender jar with a rubber spatula occasionally. Pour a third of the mixture into the bottom of a 9 × 13-inch dish, layer with half of the cookies and banana slices. Pour another third on top and layer with remaining cookies and bananas, then top with the remaining mixture, making sure to cover all of the banana slices. Sprinkle the top with crushed cookies and chill for 1 hour or if overnight, cover tightly with plastic wrap.

Variation

Add a pint of thinly sliced strawberries along with bananas.

HARVEST PIES

THERE ARE SOME FLAVORS in the world of pie that forever remind us of cool autumn days surrounded by friends and family, or just relishing a piece of pie and watching the leaves turn: warm spices, tart apples, sweet pumpkin, and rich, creamy sweet potatoes. From old-fashioned Apple Brown Betty to a creamy almond pear tart to classic pumpkin pie, these recipes are fall-themed favorites that are great any time of year. Who says you can't have a taste of October in August?

COSMOS APPLE PIE

MAKES 8 SERVINGS

If you wish to create an apple pie from scratch, you must first create the universe.
— CARL SAGAN

THIS APPLE PIE is an homage to Carl Sagan, so relish it while you gaze out into the cosmos and think about how amazing it all is, and how amazing apple pie all is.

This is probably the first pie you'll want to master and luckily it's also one of the easiest. We like to use Granny Smiths here, since they hold their shape and are tart enough to complement the sweetness and spices. The apples are perfectly plump and juicy and the luscious saucy filling just bursts all over your taste buds. A little dusting of cinnamon sugar makes the pie look and taste great. Thank you, universe!

1 recipe **OLIVE OIL DOUBLE CRUST** (page 39)
or **BUTTERY DOUBLE CRUST** (page 37),
rolled out and fit into a 9-inch pie plate

FILLING:
  6 cups peeled Granny Smith apples,
    sliced ¼ inch thick (about 3 pounds)
  ⅓ cup brown sugar
  ½ cup white sugar
  1 teaspoon ground cinnamon

  ½ teaspoon ground ginger
  ⅛ teaspoon ground cloves
  3 tablespoons all-purpose flour
  Pinch of salt

TOPPING:
  ½ teaspoon ground cinnamon
  2 tablespoons sugar
  2 tablespoons plain almond milk or
    nondairy milk of your choice

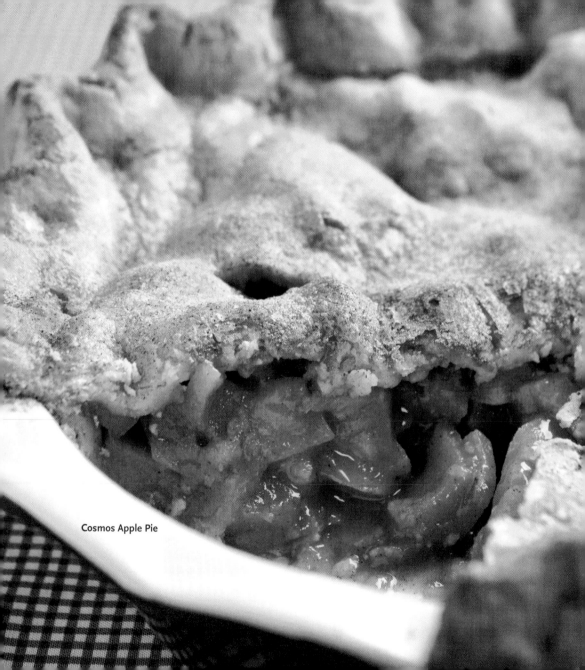

Cosmos Apple Pie

1. Combine all the filling ingredients in a large mixing bowl, tossing with your hands to coat the apples.
2. Preheat the oven to 425°F. Add the filling to the prepared pie shell. Cover with the top crust, pinch the edges together, trim the excess dough to about an inch, and crimp.
3. Mix together the cinnamon and sugar for the topping and pour the almond milk in a small cup. Brush the top of the pie with the almond milk and then sprinkle with the cinnamon sugar. Make five slits in the middle of the pie to let steam escape (a steak knife works great for this).
4. Bake the pie for 25 minutes, then lower the heat and bake for 30 to 35 more minutes, slipping on a pie crust shield if your edges are getting too browned. Place the pie on a cooling rack and let it cool for about half an hour before serving.

APPLE CREAM RAISIN PIE

MAKES ONE 10-INCH PIE

THERE'S APPLE PIE, there are creamy pies, and even pies with crumbly toppings, but all three fabulous things can be yours at once in this decadent fruit pie. It's piled high with thinly sliced tart apples and raisins that seem to melt together into the bewitching cashew-based cream.

For best results, use a 10-inch wide, deep-dish ceramic pie plate (at least 3 inches deep) to secure this plentiful crumb topping and bubbling apple goodness.

1 recipe **SINGLE (AND LOVING IT!) PASTRY CRUST** (page 42), fit into a 10-inch pie plate

TOPPING:

½ cup all-purpose flour

⅓ cup brown sugar

2 tablespoons chopped walnuts

½ teaspoon ground cinnamon

¼ teaspoon salt

6 tablespoons cold nonhydrogenated margarine

FILLING:

½ cup whole unroasted cashews, soaked in water for 2 to 8 hours or until very soft

3 tablespoons lemon juice

¼ cup soy yogurt; plain, lemon, or vanilla flavor

3 tablespoons all-purpose flour

¾ cup sugar

½ teaspoon pure vanilla extract

¾ teaspoon ground cinnamon

½ teaspoon ground ginger

½ teaspoon ground nutmeg

Pinch of salt

2½ pounds Granny Smith or any tart, firm apple

⅔ cup raisins, dark or golden

1. Preheat the oven to 425°F. Prepare the crumb topping: In a small bowl stir together the flour, brown sugar, walnuts, cinnamon, and salt. Cut 2 tablespoons of the margarine into ¼-inch cubes and reserve in the refrigerator. Use a fork or pastry cutter to cut in the remaining 4 tablespoons of the margarine until the mixture resembles fine crumbs; set aside and prepare the filling next.

2. Drain the cashews and blend with the lemon juice, soy yogurt, and flour until smooth, then use a rubber spatula to scrape the mixture into a large mixing bowl. Stir in the sugar, vanilla extract, cinnamon, ginger, nutmeg, and salt. Peel the apples, remove the cores, and slice the apples 1/8 inch thick (or as thin as you can get them using a knife). In a large mixing bowl, fold together the apples, raisins, and cashew mixture to coat the apples.

3. Spread the filling evenly into the crust and firmly pack down the apples; this is tall pie! Sprinkle generously with crumb topping and dot top with the reserved cold margarine pieces.

4. Cover top of pie tightly with foil and bake for 20 minutes, then turn heat down to 350°F and continue baking for 45 to 55 minutes, until the filling is bubbling on the edges of the pie. Remove the foil for the last 20 minutes of baking to let the crumb topping turn golden brown. (Place a pie crust shield on the edges of the pie to prevent excessive browning.) If necessary—say your deep-dish plate isn't quite deep enough—to prevent juices spilling onto the bottom of your oven, place a large rimmed baking sheet on the lower rack beneath the pie as it bakes. Let the pie cool for 25 minutes before slicing with a thin, sharp knife.

APPLE BROWN BETTY

MAKES 6 TO 8 SERVINGS

APPLE BROWN BETTY IS A HOMEY CONCOCTION of buttery breadcrumbs layered with tender, spiced apples. Casual and funky retro, this Betty is like your best friend who's at home in both combat boots and a vintage tea dress. Regular sandwich bread makes ideal crumbs, or a soft, light whole wheat bread can add a wholesome flair to this unpretentious cobbler-like dessert. For best results, use sliced bread that's a little past its prime for firmer, easy-to-toast breadcrumbs.

6 slices soft sandwich bread, about 2⅓ generous cups of crumbs

6 tablespoons nonhydrogenated margarine, divided and kept cold

3 tablespoons brown sugar

2 pounds Granny Smith or other tart baking apples

2 tablespoons fresh lemon juice

⅔ cup sugar

1 teaspoon ground cinnamon

½ teaspoon ground ginger

¼ teaspoon ground nutmeg

1. Preheat the oven to 400°F. In a food processor, pulse the bread into fine crumbs. In a large skillet melt 3 tablespoons of the margarine over medium heat. Stir in the breadcrumbs. Toast the crumbs, spreading them out in the bottom of the pan and stirring frequently, until they are golden and fragrant, about 8 to 10 minutes. Turn off the heat and stir the brown sugar into the crumbs.

2. Peel and core the apples, then cut into ¼-inch thick slices. In a large mixing bowl, toss together the apples, lemon juice, sugar, cinnamon, ginger, nutmeg, raisins, and 2 tablespoons of the breadcrumb mixture.

3. Lightly rub an 11 × 7-inch baking dish or 10-inch pie plate with a lit-

tle softened margarine and sprinkle a third of the breadcrumbs on the bottom. Layer with half the apples, top with another third of crumbs, add the remaining apple layer, and sprinkle the top evenly with the rest of the crumbs. Dot the top with the remaining 3 tablespoons of margarine cut into small pieces. Cover the dish with foil and crimp the edges tightly.

4. Bake the Betty for 35 minutes, then reduce the heat to 350°F, remove the foil, and continue baking for another 10 minutes or until the apples look juicy and the crumbs are golden brown. Let cool 10 minutes and serve warm with any whipped topping or vegan ice cream.

Variation

Add ½ cup dried cranberries. Replace ⅓ cup of the sugar with pure maple syrup.

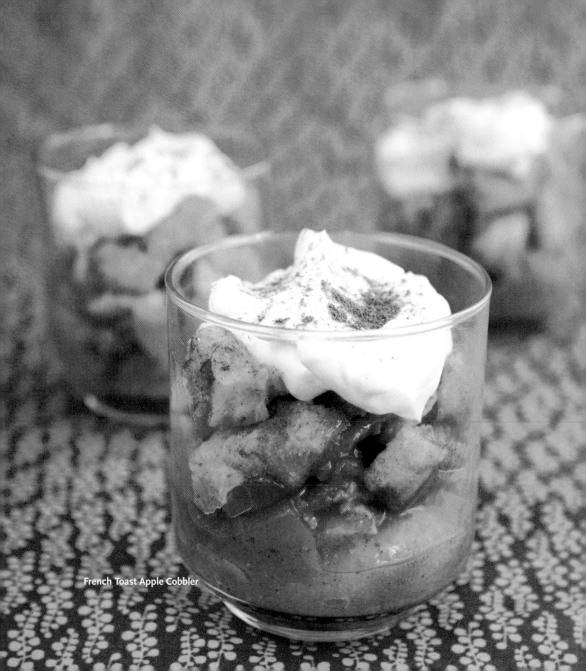

French Toast Apple Cobbler

FRENCH TOAST APPLE COBBLER

MAKES 6 TO 8 SERVINGS

OUR TESTERS WENT BANANAS (or apples?) for this hearty fusion of chewy-top, soft-underneath bread pudding and apple cobbler that happily blurs the line between dessert and brunch. If serving for brunch, consider using a soft whole wheat bread; if it's purely dessert, opt for a light, sweet white bread or even slices from a cinnamon-raisin loaf.

TOPPING:

½ cup whole unroasted cashews,
soaked in water for 2 to 8 hours or
until very soft

2 cups plain soy milk

¼ cup brown sugar

2 tablespoons nonhydrogenated
margarine, melted

4 teaspoons cornstarch

1 teaspoon pure vanilla extract

½ teaspoon maple extract

¼ teaspoon ground nutmeg

½ teaspoon ground cinnamon

Pinch of salt

6 slices slightly dry, soft sandwich
bread, crusts trimmed (about 3 cups
of ½-inch cubes)

FILLING:

2½ pounds Granny Smith or other tart
baking apples

2 tablespoons lemon juice

⅔ cup sugar

2 tablespoons all-purpose flour

2 tablespoons brown sugar

1½ teaspoons ground cinnamon

FOR SPRINKLING:

2 tablespoons turbinado sugar

¼ teaspoon ground cinnamon

RAD WHIP (page 199) or store-bought
vegan whipped topping to serve
(optional)

1. Preheat the oven to 425°F. Drain the cashews and combine them in a blender with the soy milk, brown sugar, margarine, cornstarch, vanilla extract, maple extract, nutmeg, cinnamon, and salt. Blend until very smooth. Stack the bread slices two at time, slice into ½-inch cubes, and set aside.

2. Peel and core the apples and slice into ¼-inch slices. In a 9 × 13-inch, ungreased baking dish, combine the apples, lemon juice, sugar, flour, brown sugar, and cinnamon. Cover the dish tightly with foil and bake the cobbler for 25 minutes, until the apples are soft and juicy. Remove from the oven, discard the foil, and turn heat down to 350°F.

3. Scatter the bread cubes in a large mixing bowl. Pulse the soy milk mixture one more time and pour it over the cubes. Let stand for 15 minutes, occasionally stirring the cubes to absorb more of the liquid. Spread over the baked apples and pour any of the remaining soy milk mixture evenly over the cobbler.

4. Stir together the remaining ¼ teaspoon ground cinnamon and the turbinado sugar and sprinkle over the top of the cobbler. Bake at 350°F for 20 to 25 minutes until the top is golden and the apple juices are bubbling; you may want to place a baking sheet on a rack under the pan to catch any juices that might spill over. Remove the cobbler from the oven and let it cool for 20 minutes before serving warm, topped with Rad Whip or whipped topping.

APPLE CRISP

WHEN YOU HAVE an abundance of red apples (lucky you!), Apple Crisp is the perfect device for turning them into dessert. Red apples turn meltingly tender and are a perfect complement to the crisp topping. Not that we need to sell you on crisp, but it's also much easier than pie, making it perfect for a lazy autumn day when you need dessert, like, *yesterday*.

FILLING:

4 pounds red apples (like Rome or Fuji), peeled, cored, and sliced ¼ inch thick

⅓ cup light brown sugar

⅓ cup sugar

¼ cup apple juice or cider

1 tablespoon cornstarch

1 teaspoon ground cinnamon

½ teaspoon ground nutmeg

¼ teaspoon ground allspice

⅛ teaspoon ground cloves

½ cup raisins (optional)

TOPPING:

1 cup rolled oats

1 cup all-purpose flour

½ cup light brown sugar

½ teaspoon baking powder

½ teaspoon ground cinnamon

¼ teaspoon salt

⅓ cup canola oil

3 tablespoons almond milk

1 teaspoon pure vanilla extract

1. Preheat the oven to 350°F. In an 11 × 13-inch baking dish, mix together all filling ingredients, tossing with your hands to make sure the apples are coated. Then prepare the topping.

2. In a medium-size mixing bowl, combine the oats, flour, brown sugar, baking powder, cinnamon, and salt. Add the canola oil, almond milk, and vanilla extract, and mix well. Crumble the topping over the apples. Bake for 45 minutes.

3. Remove the crisp from the oven and let cool for at least 15 minutes before serving.

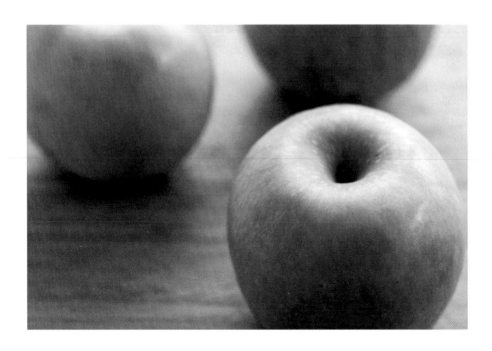

FIGGY APPLE HAND PIES

MAKES 8 HAND PIES

APPLES AND FIGS make natural companions in this hand pie that is reminiscent of a big old Fig Newton! See the Fruit Pies chapter for other hand pie recipes.

1 recipe PUFFY PIE DOUGH (page 41)

FILLING:

3 Granny Smith apples, peeled, cored, and ½-inch diced

½ pound dried black mission figs, roughly chopped

½ cup pure maple syrup

½ teaspoon ground cinnamon

Pinch of salt

2 tablespoons all-purpose flour

FOR SPRINKLING:

2 tablespoons sugar

1. After preparing the dough, divide it into two logs about 6 inches long. Wrap the logs with plastic wrap and chill for 30 to 45 minutes.

2. In the meantime, cook the filling. Combine everything in a 2-quart pot and mix well. Cover the pot and cook the apple mixture over medium heat, stirring often, for about 15 minutes, until the apples are tender and the figs have broken down and melded with the maple syrup. Let cool before filling the pastry.

3. Preheat the oven to 400°F and line two large, rimmed baking sheets with parchment paper.

4. On a lightly floured surface, roll a dough log into a roughly 14 × 7-inch rectangle. Trim the edges so that they're even. Slice the rectangle in half to form two squares. Slice the squares in half so that you have four rectangles.

5. Have a cup of water at the ready. To form the hand pie, use your fingertips dipped in water to wet the edges of a pastry rectangle. Scoop a scant ¼ cup of filling into one half of the pastry, fold it over, and quickly run your finger along the edges to press it closed. Now press a fork into the edges to create a pretty pattern and to seal the hand pie well.

6. Transfer the hand pie to a baking sheet and continue with the others. When all four pies are formed, continue with the other log of dough and place those on a separate baking sheet.

7. Brush water onto the top of each pastry and sprinkle with a little sugar. Create three slits in each hand pie to let steam escape.

8. Bake the hand pies for 30 to 35 minutes on two separate racks, switching the pans between the racks halfway through baking so that they cook evenly. The pies are ready when lightly browned at the edges and the filling is bubbly. Remove from the oven and let cool for 5 minutes. Remove the pies from the trays and let cool further. (You can just lift the parchment to move the pies to a different surface.) We like to eat them when they're still just a tiny bit warm.

PEAR FRANGIPANE TART

WHAT IS FRANGIPANE, you ask? It's a must-try style of baked almond custard filling for almond dessert fans everywhere. It's also relatively fast and easy to make in your blender, and poured over fruit and baked in a pastry crust, it puffs up golden on top with an unbeatable creamy richness beneath. It's as pretty as a French pastry shop window, and we hope you love this fragrant almond and pear tart as much as we do. Like any fruit tart this pastry has the best texture and consistency if enjoyed the day it's made.

1 recipe **SHORTBREAD TART SHELL** (page 44) or **PRESS-IN ALMOND CRUST** (page 52) fitted into a 10-inch tart pan and partially baked for 15 minutes

FILLING:

6 tablespoons cold nonhydrogenated margarine, cut into pieces

½ cup sugar

1¼ cups blanched sliced almonds, pulsed in a food processor into a fine meal

2 tablespoons cornstarch

¼ teaspoon ground cinnamon

Pinch of salt

⅔ cup almond milk

2 teaspoons pure vanilla extract

½ teaspoon almond extract

3 baking pears (Bartlett or Bosc), ripe but not overly mushy

1. Preheat the oven to 350°F. In a food processor pulse together the margarine, sugar, pulsed almonds, cornstarch, cinnamon, and salt until crumbly. Continue to pulse and stream in the almond milk, vanilla extract, and almond extract to form a thick batter. Pour this frangipane mixture into the tart shell.

2. Peel the pears, remove their cores

Pear Frangipane Tart

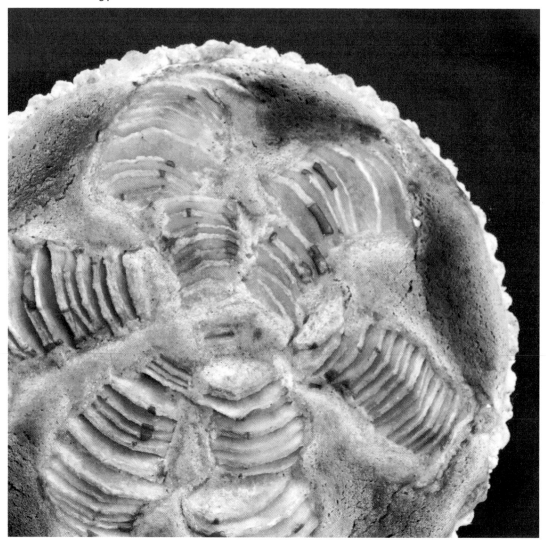

and slice each pear in half. Holding onto a pear half to help keep it together during slicing, slice each half into ¼-inch slices, and layer slices, overlapping, on top of the frangipane mixture; the pears will partially sink into the batter. For easier moving of sliced pears, slide your knife underneath the pears, press down on them gently to slightly fan them out, and then slide them into the batter.

3. Bake the tart for 40 to 42 minutes until the filling is puffed up around the pears. To further brown the top of the tart broil on high heat for 1 to 1½ minutes until the top just begins to turn golden, but watch (very!) carefully to avoid burning. Promptly remove the tart, transfer to a cooling rack, and let cool at least 2 hours before slicing with a thin, sharp knife dipped in cold water.

Slices

Once peeled, pears will brown quickly! To prevent further browning, rub peeled pears with lemon juice before slicing.

PEAR & CRANBERRY GALETTE

MAKES TWO GALETTES (8 SERVINGS)

A GALETTE IS a fancier, more French way of saying "free-form pie." We love the rustic look of this pie combined with the homey taste of buckwheat. A handful of cranberries is perfect for lending tart flavor and splashes of color to the pears; they look like a watercolor painting as they cook and burst. This galette is fabulous with vegan vanilla ice cream.

1 recipe **BUCKWHEAT DOUBLE CRUST** (page 51)

FILLING:

4 Bosc pears, peeled, thinly sliced (see tip)

½ cup brown sugar

1 teaspoon ground cinnamon

2 tablespoons all-purpose flour

Pinch of salt

½ cup whole cranberries (fresh or frozen)

1. In a large mixing bowl, mix together pears, sugar, cinnamon, flour and salt. Be gentle because pears are somewhat fragile.

2. Preheat the oven to 400°F. Line a large, rimmed baking sheet with parchment paper.

3. On a lightly floured surface, roll half the dough into a 14-inch circle. Transfer the crust to the baking sheet. It's okay if the edges droop over the baking sheet; you'll be folding them up.

4. Layer the pear mixture into the crust, leaving 2 inches clear around the edges. Start with a single layer and add a second layer from the center out when you run out of space. Fold the edges up over the filling. Sprinkle on ¼ cup of cranberries. Proceed with the

second galette, preparing it as you did the first, on the same baking sheet.

5. Make two double-layer squares of aluminum foil that are big enough to cover the open part of the galette. Loosely cover the galettes with foil; this will prevent the pears from drying out while they bake.

6. Bake the galettes for 30 minutes, then remove the foil and bake for 15 to 20 minutes more. The pears should be tender and the cranberries should be juicy and bleeding into the pears.

7. Remove the galettes from the oven and let them rest until cool enough to serve. Slice each into 4 pieces and serve.

Slices

To prepare the pears, peel them, remove the stem, and slice them in half lengthwise. Now use a teaspoon measuring spoon to scoop out the seeds; it should work like a melon baller leaving a perfectly circular cutout. Now simply slice the pears in strips that are a little less than ¼ inch thick.

SWEET POTATO BRAZIL NUT CRUNCH PIE

MAKES ONE 9-INCH PIE

A VELVETY SWEET potato pie bursting with tropical charm: coconut milk, lime, rum, allspice, and a toothsome Brazil nut crumble topping. Roasting whole sweet potatoes in their skins yields the most flavorful filling, but in a pinch you can steam or microwave peeled sweet potatoes.

1 recipe **SINGLE (AND LOVING IT!) PIE CRUST**
(page 42)

FILLING:

2 cups mashed cooked sweet potatoes
(about 1½ pounds uncooked sweet
potatoes)
1 cup plus 2 tablespoons coconut milk
3 tablespoons cornstarch
½ cup dark brown sugar
¼ cup sugar
1 tablespoon dark rum
1 tablespoon lime juice
½ teaspoon finely grated lime zest
½ teaspoon ground cinnamon
½ teaspoon ground ginger
¼ teaspoon ground allspice
¼ teaspoon salt
Pinch of ground nutmeg

TOPPING:

½ cup dark brown sugar
2 tablespoons nonhydrogenated
margarine
Pinch of salt
1 cup whole Brazil nuts, roughly
chopped

1. Preheat the oven to 350°F. Prepare the pie crust recipe as directed and blind bake for 10 minutes. Remove it from the oven and set aside.

2. In a blender, combine the filling ingredients and pulse several times until very creamy and smooth. Pour the filling into the prebaked crust and smooth out the top with a rubber spatula, tak-

ing care to leave the center slightly shallower than the edges to help the center firm up faster while baking.

3. While the pie is baking prepare the topping: In a small bowl mash together brown sugar and margarine until crumbly, then mash in chopped nuts and salt.

4. Bake the pie for 20 minutes, then remove it from the oven and sprinkle with the Brazil nut topping. Bake another 28 to 30 minutes, until the nuts look toasted and the top is bubbling. Remove the pie from the oven and let it completely cool before slicing, at least 2 hours.

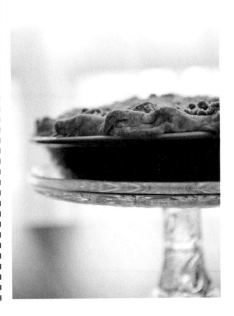

SWEET POTATO COBBLER

FOR SWEET POTATO DESSERT LOVERS, tender slices of sweet potato in a spicy syrup tucked between layers of buttery pastry sets a whole new standard. This is a citrus-kissed tribute to the classic and ultra-comforting Southern-style treat that's great for a hearty dessert or pretty brunch centerpiece.

1 recipe **BUTTERY DOUBLE CRUST** (page 37), top crust made into a lattice top

FILLING:

- 2 pounds sweet potatoes, peeled and sliced into ¼-inch slices
- ⅔ cup brown sugar
- 3 tablespoons sugar
- ⅓ cup freshly squeezed orange juice
- 1 tablespoon lemon juice
- Grated zest of 1 orange
- 1 teaspoon ground cinnamon
- 1 teaspoon ground ginger
- ⅛ teaspoon ground cloves
- 2 tablespoons cornstarch

TOPPING:

- 2 tablespoons soy milk
- 1 tablespoon turbinado sugar

1. In a large pot, cover the sweet potatoes with 3 quarts of cold water. Bring to a boil over high heat, then reduce the heat to medium. Continue to cook the potatoes until they just start to become tender enough to pierce easily with a fork but are not mushy, about 8 to 10 minutes. Set aside 2 cups of the cooking liquid and drain the rest, setting aside the potatoes.

2. Return the reserved cooking liquid to the pot. Whisk in the brown sugar, sugar, orange juice, lemon juice, orange zest, cinnamon, ginger, and cloves. Bring to a gentle boil over medium heat and cook for 10 minutes, stirring occasionally; the liquid should resemble a thin syrup. Remove the syrup from the heat and let it cool to room temperature.

3. While the syrup is cooling, preheat the oven to 425°F. Lightly oil a 10-inch ceramic deep-dish pie plate or square baking pan. Press in the bottom crust, fold in any hanging edges, and prick the crust with a fork about 30 times. Bake the crust for 12 to 14 minutes or until firm, then remove from the oven.

4. Layer the drained sweet potatoes over the bottom crust. Whisk the cornstarch into the cooled syrup and pour the syrup over the sweet potatoes. Then, top the filling with the lattice top crust and crimp the edges. Brush the top of the crust with soy milk and sprinkle it with turbinado sugar.

5. Bake the pie for 25 minutes, then reduce the heat to 350°F and bake for 25 to 30 minutes more, until the juices are thickened and bubbling through the lattice holes. Remove the pie from the oven and let cool for 20 minutes before slicing. Serve with **RAD WHIP** (page 199) or vegan vanilla ice cream.

Variation

Stir 1 cup drained juice-packed crushed pineapple into the liquid ingredients before pouring over the sweet potatoes.

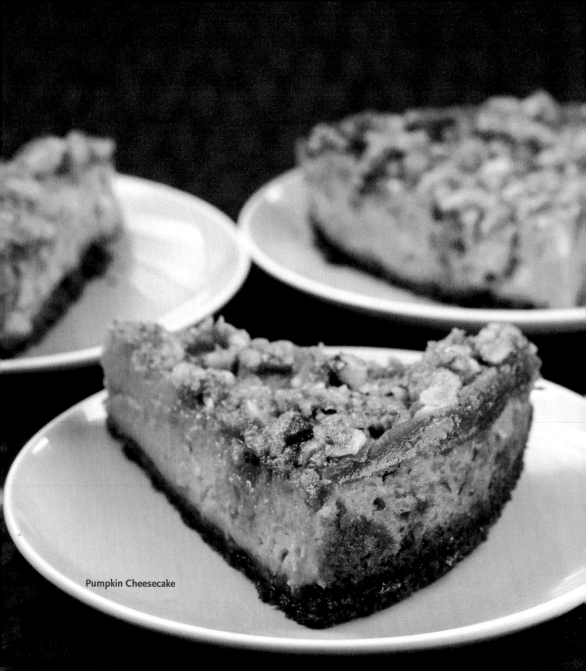

Pumpkin Cheesecake

PUMPKIN CHEESECAKE

PUMPKIN CHEESECAKE: two words that always get our attention, and likely yours as well. While fresh pumpkin is great for straight-up pies, we prefer the consistency and flavor of canned for this insanely popular fall-time dessert; plus canned pumpkin equals pumpkin cheesecake all year round. See tip on page 94 for crack-free cheesecake baking!

1 recipe **GRAHAM CRACKER CRUST** (page 46), or Vanilla Cookie Crust variation

FILLING:

½ cup whole unroasted cashews, soaked in water for 2 to 8 hours or until very soft

¼ cup mashed banana (about 1 medium-size banana)

1 (12–14 ounce) package silken tofu, drained

½ cup sugar

⅓ cup dark brown sugar

3 tablespoons coconut oil, room temperature

6 teaspoons cornstarch

2 tablespoons lemon juice

2½ teaspoons pure vanilla extract

¼ teaspoon orange extract or 1 teaspoon grated orange zest

¼ teaspoon sea salt

1¼ cups canned pumpkin puree

¾ teaspoon ground cinnamon

½ teaspoon ground ginger

¼ teaspoon ground nutmeg

TOPPING:

⅓ cup brown sugar

1 tablespoon nonhydrogenated margarine

Pinch of salt

1 cup pecan pieces, roughly chopped

1. Make the topping first. In a mixing bowl use a fork to mash together brown sugar, margarine and salt until crumbly, then fold in the chopped nuts and stir to coat with the mixture. Set aside until ready to use.

2. Preheat the oven to 350°F and lightly spray the bottom and sides of a 9-inch springform pan with nonstick cooking spray. Prepare the crust and press it very firmly into the bottom of the pan. Bake for 10 minutes and move the pan to a cooling rack, leaving the oven on for further baking in a bit.

3. Meanwhile, prepare the filling: Drain the cashews and blend with the banana, tofu, sugar, brown sugar, coconut oil, cornstarch, lemon juice, vanilla and orange extracts, and sea salt. Blend until completely smooth and no bits of cashew remain.

4. Set aside ⅓ cup of batter. To the remaining batter, add the pumpkin puree, cinnamon, ginger, and nutmeg and blend until smooth, then pour it onto the crust. Randomly spoon dollops of the reserved batter onto the cheesecake. Poke the end of a chopstick into a batter blob and gently swirl to create a marble pattern; repeat with the remaining plain dollops.

5. Bake the cheesecake for 45 to 50 minutes. Remove cheesecake halfway through baking and sprinkle on the topping. Return to oven to continue baking. Cheesecake will be done when the top is lightly puffed and the edges of the cake are golden. Remove it from the oven and let cool on a rack for 20 minutes, then transfer to the fridge to complete cooling, at least 3 hours or even better, overnight. To serve, slice the cake using a thin, sharp knife dipped in cold water.

KITTEE'S SWEET POTATO HAND PIES

MAKES 8 HAND PIES

HAND PIES ARE a giant, ubiquitous institution in New Orleans. They come in lots of flavors, even seasonal ones like sweet potato and strawberry, but are typically made with lard-filled dough. Here's a vegan sweet potato version from our crafty pal Kittee that looks just like the kind you'll find in Nola! If you like, coat these hand pies in glaze and sprinkle with colorful cinnamon sugar.

1 recipe PUFFY PIE DOUGH (page 41)

FILLING:
 2 cups mashed sweet potato flesh, cooled (from 2 small-medium sweet potatoes, baked, see tip)
 1½ tablespoons cornstarch
 ¾ teaspoon ground cinnamon
 ⅛ teaspoon ground allspice
 ⅓ cup sugar
 2 teaspoons fresh grated ginger
 Dash of salt, to taste

GLAZE:
 2 tablespoons almond milk
 1 cup confectioner's sugar, sifted
 ¼ teaspoon pure vanilla extract

OPTIONAL:
 Colorful decorating sugar

1. In a medium-size mixing bowl, mix all the filling ingredients together, mashing well with a fork.
2. Preheat the oven to 400°F and line two large, rimmed baking sheets with parchment paper.
3. On a lightly floured surface, roll a dough log into a roughly 14 × 7-inch rectangle. Trim the edges with a paring knife so that they're even. Slice the rectangle in half to form two squares. Slice the squares in half so that you have four rectangles.

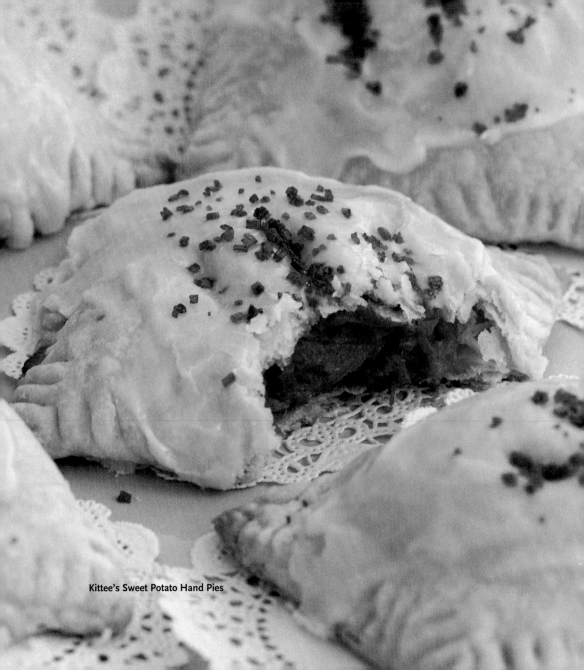

Kittee's Sweet Potato Hand Pies

4. To form the hand pie, use your fingertips dipped in water to wet the edges of a pastry rectangle. Scoop a scant ¼ cup of filling into one half of the pastry and fold it over, quickly running your finger along the edges to press them closed. Now press a fork into the edges to create a pretty crimped pattern and to seal the hand pie well.

5. Transfer the hand pie to a baking sheet and continue with the others. When all four pies are formed, continue with the other log of dough and place those on a separate baking sheet. Create three slits in each hand pie to let steam escape.

6. Bake for 25 minutes on two separate racks, switching the pans between racks halfway through baking so that they cook evenly. The pies are ready when lightly browned at the edges. Remove them from the oven and let cool for 5 minutes. Remove the pies from the trays and let cool completely. (You can just lift the parchment to transfer the pies to a different surface.)

7. When pies are still a little bit warm, prepare the glaze by vigorously mixing the ingredients together. The consistency should be pretty drippy but not watery. If it seems too stiff, add a smidge more almond milk. Use a spoon to coat each pie with glaze. To prevent a big mess, just place your cooling rack right over the sink to catch the excess glaze. Sprinkle liberally with decorating sugar, if using.

8. Continue to let the hand pies cool. If the glaze still seems sticky, place the pies in the freezer for 5 minutes to make it set.

✳ *Slices* ✳

To prepare mashed sweet potato, preheat the oven to 350°F and place sweet potatoes directly on the oven rack. Bake for about 50 minutes, let cool, peel, and mash away!

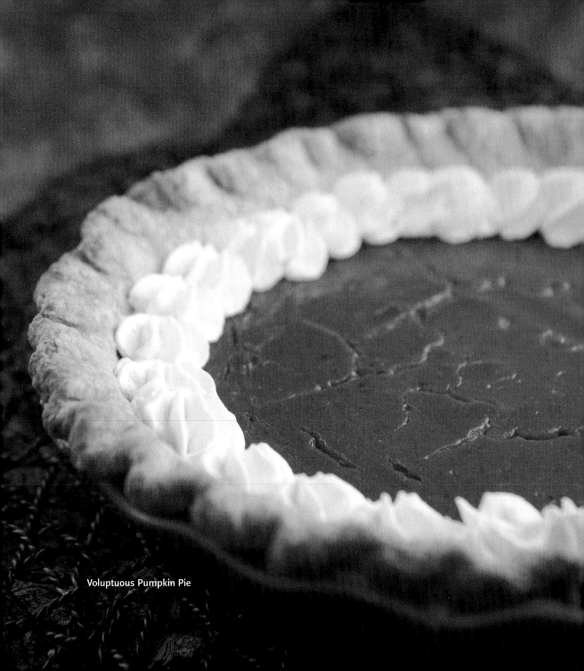

Voluptuous Pumpkin Pie

VOLUPTUOUS PUMPKIN PIE

MAKES ONE 9-INCH PIE

WHY MESS WITH PERFECTION? Myra Kornfeld invented the perfect vegan pumpkin pie recipe in her 2000 cookbook *The Voluptuous Vegan*, and it's been our go-to ever since. We're proud to present a slightly modified version of her recipe that tastes great made either with freshly roasted fall pumpkin or canned pumpkin. It's custardy, spicy, not too sweet, and everything you want in a forkful of pumpkin pie.

1 recipe **SINGLE (AND LOVING IT!) PASTRY CRUST** (page 42), fit into a 9-inch pie plate

FILLING:
  3 cups pumpkin puree (canned or fresh) or other sweet winter squash
  ½ cup pure maple syrup
  ½ cup plain unsweetened soy milk
  4 teaspoons canola oil
  1 teaspoon ground cinnamon
  1 teaspoon ground ginger
  ¼ teaspoon ground nutmeg
  Pinch of ground cloves
  ½ teaspoon salt
  2 tablespoons cornstarch
  1 teaspoon agar powder

1. Preheat the oven to 350°F. In a blender, pulse together the pumpkin, maple syrup, soy milk, canola oil, cinnamon, ginger, nutmeg, cloves, salt, cornstarch, and agar powder until very smooth. Pour the filling into the pie shell.

2. Bake the pie for 60 to 65 minutes, until the center looks semi-firm, not liquidy. Check the edges of the crust after baking for 40 minutes; if the edges appear to be browning too rapidly, carefully remove the pie and apply crust protectors to the edges to keep the crust from getting too dark.

⋆ ⋆ ⋆

ROASTING FRESH PUMPKIN

PREPARING FRESH PUMPKINS (or any sweet winter squash) for pies is as easy as turning on your oven. For best flavor, save the really big pumpkins for jack-o'-lanterns or curries and use small sugar pumpkins that have firmly attached stems and feel heavy for their size. A small, 2- to 2 ½-pound pumpkin will provide plenty of cooked pumpkin for one 9-inch pie.

1. Preheat the oven to 425°F and have ready a large, rimmed baking sheet.
2. Slice the pumpkin in half, crosswise, scoop out the seeds and stringy bits, and wrap each cut half tightly with foil. Place foil sides down on sheet; make sure to use only a rimmed sheet as the baking pumpkin will produce plenty of juice as it bakes.
3. Bake for 35 to 45 minutes until a sharp knife can be easily inserted through the pumpkin and the flesh is very soft. Let cool long enough to scoop out the flesh and roughly mash in a mixing bowl. To measure, firmly pack the pumpkin flesh into a measuring cup.
4. If the pumpkin flesh seems really watery, you may want to drain it before measuring. Scoop the flesh into a fine mesh metal strainer and let it sit over a bowl for an hour or more until the desired consistency is reached. Or, if you want to get it done faster and have some cheesecloth lying around, you can wrap the pumpkin flesh tightly in the cloth and squeeze out the excess water.

3. Remove the pie from the oven and transfer it onto a cooling rack for 30 minutes, then chill for at least 4 hours before slicing. Serve with **RAD WHIP** (page 199), vegan whipped topping, or your favorite vegan vanilla ice cream. In the photo, we piped cream around the edges of the pie with a large decorating tip; try it yourself when presenting the pie to your pumpkin pie–loving guests.

MAPLE PECAN PIE

MAKES ONE 9-INCH PIE OR ONE 11-INCH TART

THIS IS THE KIND of pecan pie that has pecans resting in a sweet suspension, somewhere between gel and custard. We're not going to make any apologies for the tofu in it . . . it works! This pie flies off the table at bake sales and makes even the most un-vegan Southerners weep with joy. Well, we *think* it's joy.

1 recipe **SINGLE PASTRY CRUST** (page 42), fit into a 9-inch pie plate

FILLING:
- ½ cup sugar
- ½ cup brown sugar
- ½ cup pure maple syrup
- ¼ cup nonhydrogenated margarine
- 6 ounces extra-firm silken tofu (½ of a tetra pack)
- ¼ cup cold unsweetened plain nondairy milk
- 2 tablespoons cornstarch
- ½ teaspoon salt
- 1 teaspoon pure vanilla extract
- 2 cups pecan halves

1. First we're going to make a caramel. In a 2-quart saucepan, mix together the sugars and the maple syrup. Heat over medium heat, stirring often with a whisk. Once small bubbles start rapidly forming, stir pretty constantly for about 10 minutes. The mixture should become thick and syrupy. It shouldn't be boiling too fiercely; if big bubbles start climbing the walls of the pan then lower the heat a bit.

2. Add the margarine and stir to melt. Turn the heat off, transfer the mixture to a mixing bowl, and let it cool for a bit. In the meantime, prepare the rest of the filling.

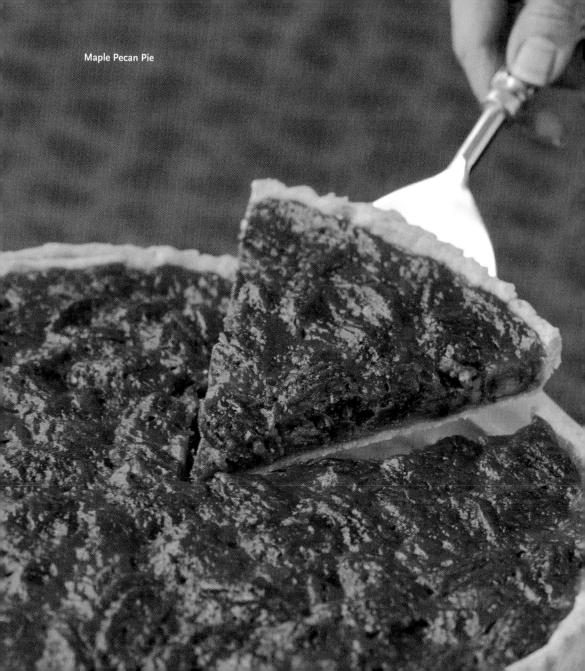

Maple Pecan Pie

3. Crumble the tofu into a blender or food processor, along with the milk, cornstarch, and salt. Puree until completely smooth, scraping down the sides of the blender to make sure you get everything.

4. Preheat the oven to 350°F. Check to see that the sugar mixture has cooled sufficiently; it's okay if it's a bit warm, just not boiling hot. Add the tofu mixture and the vanilla extract to the sugar mixture and mix well. Fold in the pecans to incorporate.

5. Transfer the filling to the prepared pie crust and bake for 40 minutes. When done, the pie is going to be somewhat jiggly, but it should appear to be set. Let cool, slice, and serve! No cheating and pulling pecans off the pie.

Variation

SALTED MAPLE PECAN PIE: Sprinkle ½ teaspoon coarse sea salt over the cooled pie.

Slices

This pie works great in tart form, too (as in the photo). Just press the crust into an 11-inch tart pan and proceed with the recipe.

CURRIED MACAROON PIE

WE ARE IN LOVE with curry desserts, and if you are, too, you will be in love with this pie. Shredded coconut in a thick and gooey caramel macaroon, turned vibrant and golden with curry powder. It may sound a little strange to you, but live a little and give it a shot!

1 recipe GINGERSNAP CRUST (page 48)

FILLING:

8 ounces unsweetened shredded
    coconut
1 cup coconut milk, divided
3 tablespoons cornstarch
½ cup brown rice syrup
½ cup brown sugar
¼ teaspoon salt
1 tablespoon mild curry powder

1. Preheat the oven to 350°F. Bake the crust for 10 minutes and remove it from the oven. Place the coconut in a mixing bowl and set aside.

2. In a saucepot, vigorously mix together ½ cup of the coconut milk and the cornstarch using a fork, until the cornstarch is dissolved. Mix in the brown rice syrup, sugar, salt, and curry powder.

3. Now you'll make a caramel. Bring the mixture to a low boil and then lower the heat to simmer for about 5 minutes, stirring occasionally. Tiny bubbles should be forming quickly and the mixture should be thickening slightly.

4. Transfer the caramel to the mixing bowl with the coconut and add in the remaining ½ cup of coconut milk. Mix well. Transfer the caramel-coconut mixture to the pie crust. Bake the pie for 25 minutes, then remove and cool completely. Slice into eighths and serve.

Slices

If you are using a very spicy curry powder, you may want to reduce it to 2 teaspoons.

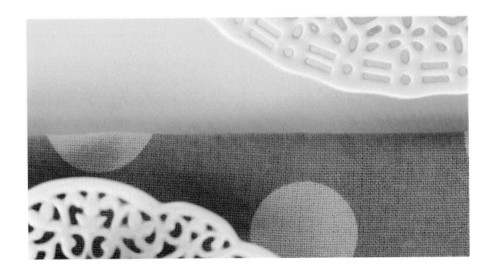

CHOCOLATE PIES

SOME PEOPLE FEEL that if you haven't had chocolate, you haven't had dessert. Who are we to argue? It's a basic human sweet-tooth need, expressed perfectly when served in a pie crust and then enhanced with caramel, fruits, nuts, and creamy fillings. When in doubt, a chocolaty cheesecake or an old-fashioned chocolate pudding pie is always a revered after-dinner guest.

OLD-FASHIONED CHOCOLATE PUDDING PIE

MAKES ONE 9-INCH PIE

YOU KNOW HOW vegan recipes are always like "This ain't your grandma's puddin' pie!" Well, this *is* your grandma's puddin' pie, only it's vegan! Smooth, cool, and creamy pudding in a classic graham cracker shell. To make life even easier, you have our permission to use store-bought crust here. For added grandma love, serve with vegan whipped cream and shaved chocolate.

1 recipe GRAHAM CRACKER CRUST (page 46), or use a store-bought 9-inch vegan graham cracker crust

FILLING:

3 cups almond milk

¼ cup cornstarch

⅓ cup sugar

3 tablespoons unsweetened cocoa powder

Big pinch of salt

¼ cup semisweet chocolate chips

1 teaspoon pure vanilla extract

1. Preheat the oven to 350°F. Bake the crust for 10 minutes, remove it from the oven, and let cool.

2. In a small (2-quart) saucepan off the heat, combine 1 cup of the almond milk and the cornstarch. Use a fork to whisk it until the cornstarch is good and dissolved. Whisk in the remaining almond milk, the sugar, cocoa powder, and salt. It's okay if the cocoa is a bit clumpy at first; it will dissolve eventually.

3. Bring the mixture to a boil, whisking occasionally. Keep a close eye because once boiling, you want to lower the heat and bring it to a slow rolling boil. Whisk consistently until the mixture is thickened, which should be about 7 minutes.

4. Add the chocolate chips and mix

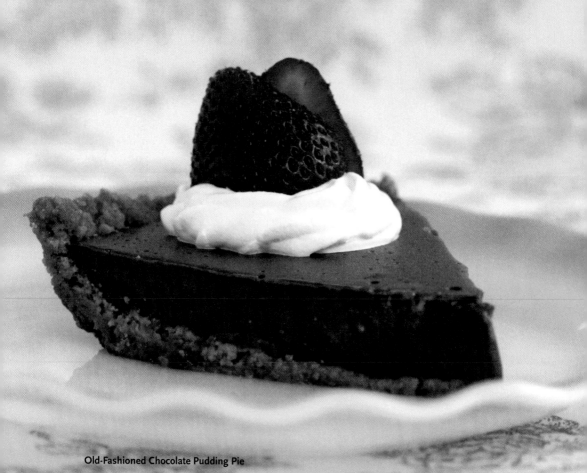

Old-Fashioned Chocolate Pudding Pie

to melt. Stir in the vanilla extract. Pour the pudding into the prepared pie shell and let cool for about 15 minutes on the counter, just until it stops steaming like mad. To keep a skin from forming, place a circle of parchment paper over the filling. Refrigerate and let set for at least 3 hours.

Variation

S'MORES PIE: Mound the pie with RAD WHIP (page 199) or vegan whipped topping, drizzle with CHOCOLATE DRIZZLE (page 203), and crumble eight graham crackers over the top.

Slices

If you're making your own crust here, use a shallow pie pan rather than a deep dish.

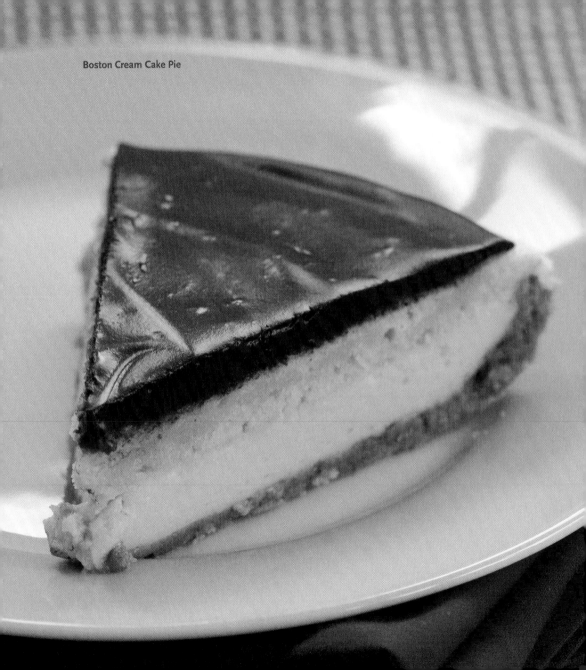
Boston Cream Cake Pie

BOSTON CREAM CAKE PIE

THIS CAKE DISGUISED AS PIE is actually a clever layering of dark chocolate ganache, white cake, and smooth vanilla cream nestled in a buttery cookie crust. Serve in Boston, Brooklyn, or Baltimore, wherever you take this "pybrid" dessert they'll be impressed with each pretty stratified slice. Or top with bright-colored sprinkles and a birthday candle and go thrill someone special with our favorite variation, Birthday Cake Pie.

1 recipe **GRAHAM CRACKER CRUST** (page 46), using either the Chocolate Cookie Crust or Vanilla Cookie Crust variation, unbaked (don't press it into the pan yet!)

CAKE LAYER:
½ cup all-purpose flour
1 tablespoon cornstarch
½ teaspoon baking powder
⅛ teaspoon salt
¾ cup plain soy milk
½ teaspoon apple cider vinegar
3 tablespoons sugar
2 tablespoons canola oil
1 teaspoon pure vanilla extract

VANILLA CRÈME LAYER:
6 ounces silken tofu, drained (half a box of Mori-Nu brand)
Generous pinch of salt
1 teaspoon pure vanilla extract
½ teaspoon lemon juice
⅛ teaspoon almond extract
1 cup soy milk
½ teaspoon agar powder
½ cup sugar
1 tablespoon cornstarch
2 tablespoons coconut oil, room temperature

GANACHE:

⅓ cup soy milk

¾ cup semisweet chocolate chips

2 tablespoons nonhydrogenated margarine

1. First, prepare the cake layer. Preheat the oven to 350°F and generously spray a 9-inch pie plate with nonstick cooking spray.

2. Sift together the flour, cornstarch, baking powder, and salt in a mixing bowl and form a well in the center. In a large measuring cup, whisk together the soy milk, apple cider vinegar, sugar, oil, and vanilla extract until smooth. Pour this mixture into the dry ingredients and use a rubber spatula to stir just until the ingredients are moistened.

3. Transfer the batter to the pie dish, smooth out the top, and bake for 12 to 14 minutes, or until a toothpick inserted into the center of the cake comes out mostly clean (a few crumbs is fine). The cake may look shiny on top, and that's okay! Place the pie plate on a cooling rack and let cool for 5 minutes.

4. Now we're going to invert the cake. Place a large dinner plate over the cake, put on your oven mitts, grab the pie plate and dish, and flip it over. Tap the bottom of the pie dish a few times to help release the cake onto the plate. Cover the warm cake with plastic wrap and set it aside.

5. Wash the pie plate, wipe it dry, and generously spray it with nonstick cooking spray. Press the cookie crust mixture into the dish (see page 46 for detailed instructions) and bake for 10 minutes. Remove the crust from the oven and let it cool while you're making the rest of the pie. You're halfway there!

6. Now we'll make the cream filling. In a blender, combine the tofu, salt, vanilla extract, lemon juice, and almond extract. Let it sit there for a moment while we work on the rest.

7. In a small saucepan, combine ½ cup of the soy milk and the agar

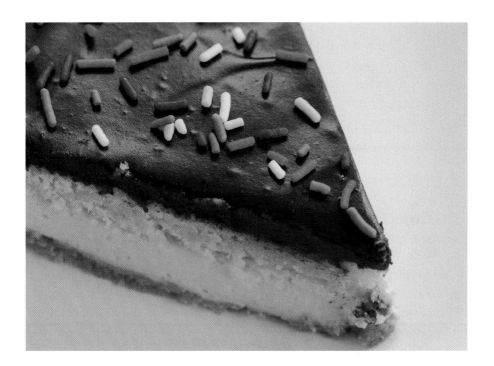

powder. Bring mixture to a boil over medium-high heat and cook for 30 seconds, reduce the heat to a simmer and cook for 5 minutes, stirring occasionally. Stir in the sugar.

8. In a measuring cup, whisk together the remaining ½ cup of soy milk and the cornstarch. Slowly pour this into the simmering soy milk mixture and stir constantly until thickened, about 5 minutes. Add the coconut oil and stir until melted.

9. Scrape this cooked mixture into the blender with the tofu. Puree until everything is very smooth, scraping the sides of the blender jar with a rubber spatula occasionally. Immediately pour the

hot cream filling into the baked pie shell. Tap the pie plate a few times to bring any air bubbles to the surface. Chill the pie for 10 minutes to help speed the setting of the filling.

10. When the filling feels slightly firmer to the touch, unwrap the inverted cake layer and carefully slide it onto the pie so that it's centered on top of the filling.

11. Now prepare the ganache topping—you're in the home stretch! In a small saucepan, bring the soy milk to a rapid simmer for 1 minute over medium heat. Turn off the flame and use a rubber spatula to stir in the chocolate chips and margarine. Continue to stir until the chips are completely melted and the mixture is very smooth. Pour the ganache onto the center of the cake and use a spatula to spread it over the top of the cake, leaving a sliver of cake exposed around the circumference.

12. Return the cake to the refrigerator once more to chill completely, at least 3 hours or even better, overnight. To serve, slice with a thin, sharp knife dipped in cold water, wiping the knife clean after each slice.

✳ *Slices* ✳

Please note that this recipe has several steps that are best made in the order listed; no need to freak out, just read the entire recipe thoroughly and take your time. To make your workflow more efficient, prepare the cookie crust mixture and have it ready in a mixing bowl; when the cake layer is done, clean the pie plate, press in the crust and bake as directed on page 46.

LAGUSTA'S CHOCOLATE RASPBERRY TART

MAKES ONE 10-INCH TART

RASPBERRY AND CHOCOLATE LOVERS, UNITE! This is basically a truffle made into a tart, studded with delicious fruity raspberries. It's so insanely rich that the tiniest sliver is really all you need, making it the perfect choice for a large party because one tart can give you 16 or more slices. The recipe comes from our favorite chocolatier, Lagusta of Lagusta's Luscious. You can order her chocolates online (www.lagustasluscious.com) or check out her 100 percent vegan chocolate shop in Poughkeepsie, New York.

1 recipe **SHORTBREAD TART SHELL** (page 44) or **PRESS-IN ALMOND CRUST** (page 52), fit into a 10-inch tart pan, baked and cooled

FILLING:

¾ cup coconut milk

2 tablespoons coconut oil

2 tablespoons water

1 cup semisweet chocolate chips

1 cup raspberries

Extra raspberries for garnish

1. In a small (2-quart) saucepot, bring the coconut milk, coconut oil, and water to a rolling boil.

2. Place the chocolate chips in a mixing bowl. In a separate small bowl, mash the raspberries into small pieces with a fork.

3. When the coconut milk mixture comes to a boil, remove it from the heat and pour it over the chocolate. Cover the bowl with a plate or lid and let sit for five minutes. Then, whisk this mixture together to create a thick ganache. Fold in the raspberries.

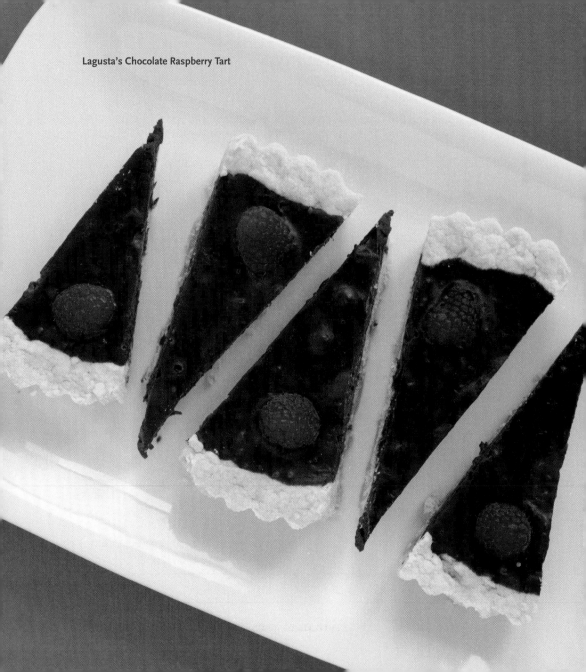

Lagusta's Chocolate Raspberry Tart

4. Pour the ganache into the baked tart shell. Smooth with a knife or spatula, if needed. Let chill for at least 2 hours before cutting. If you like, add fresh raspberries to the circumference of the crust to decorate it.

5. Slice the tart into 16 thin slices, dipping a knife into warm water and wiping it clean after each cut.

Slices

Thawed frozen raspberries will work well for the tart filling, but use only fresh for the garnish. If you have no fresh ones, just skip the garnish completely. It will still be beautiful!

CHOCOLATE HAZELNUT TRUFFLE TART

MAKES 16 SERVINGS

REMINISCENT OF CHOCOLATE HAZELNUT SPREAD, this decadent and luscious pie is a serious crowd pleaser. Like standing ovation, throw-roses-on-the-stage crowd pleaser. Each slice is so rich that a sliver will do you just fine.

1 recipe **SHORTBREAD TART SHELL** (page 44) or **PRESS-IN ALMOND CRUST** (page 52), fit into a 10-inch tart pan, baked and cooled

FILLING:

1½ cups hazelnuts

¾ cup coconut milk

1½ cups semisweet chocolate chips

1 teaspoon pure vanilla extract

1. Preheat the oven to 325°F. Spread the hazelnuts out in a single layer on a rimmed baking sheet. Toast the hazelnuts for 10 to 15 minutes, tossing them about halfway through. Remove from the oven and place the nuts on a clean kitchen towel. Wrap up the towel and rub the nuts (snicker) together vigorously to remove the skins. You don't have to be too meticulous about this; some skins remaining are okay.

2. Place 1¼ cups of the hazelnuts in a food processor and set the remaining ¼ cup aside. Grind the hazelnuts into a crunchy nut butter—this could take 5 to 7 minutes—scraping down the sides of the bowl often. It doesn't have to be totally smooth, but it should be a paste. Add a tablespoon or 2 of water if needed, to get the nuts to blend better.

3. In the meantime, bring the coconut milk to a boil in a small saucepot. Place the chocolate chips in a large bowl. Once the coconut milk

I'LL MELT WITH YOU, CHOCOLATE

FOR YEARS, WE WERE RESISTANT to using a microwave to melt chocolate, but we've given in because it's just too easy! To melt chocolate in a microwave, place the chips in a microwave-safe bowl and heat in the microwave for 45 seconds. Remove the bowl and use a fork to give the chips a stir. If they are very melty, heat them again for only another 20 seconds. If they are not at all melty, give them another 45 seconds. Remove from microwave once again, and give them a stir. At this point they should be mostly melted, so just stir in order to get them thoroughly smooth and melted.

To melt chocolate on the stove top, you'll need a small pot of boiling water, and another small, shallow pan to put on top of that. Place the chocolate chips in the pan on top of the boiling water, and give them a minute to get melty. Once melty, stir with a rubber spatula until thoroughly melted.

is boiling, pour it over the chocolate chips. Cover the bowl with a plate and let sit for 5 minutes. Mix it with a fork until smooth, then mix in the hazelnut butter and vanilla extract.

4. Spread the mixture into the baked tart shell. Top with the remaining hazelnuts and let chill for at least 2 hours, or until set. To serve, slice the tart into 16 thin slices, dipping the knife into warm water and wiping clean after each cut.

CHOCOLATE-ORANGE HAZELNUT TARTS

MAKES SIX 4-INCH TARTS

OUR FAVORITE CHOCOLATE-OLIVE OIL CRUST cradles this delicate creamy filling spiked with orange, hazelnut, chocolate ganache, and a hint of coffee. It's a flavor marriage that's totally Spanish and will make you feel like you're strolling down La Rambla in Barcelona with every chocolate-orange-hazelnut-coffee bite.

Coffee extract is essential here; it won't tint the color of the filling and lends just the right amount of coffee flavor.

1 recipe CHOCOLATE OLIVE OIL SHORTBREAD CRUST (page 49), fit into six 4-inch tart shells, baked and cooled (see page 177)

FILLING:
- ½ cup whole unroasted cashews, soaked in water for 2 to 8 hours or until very soft
- ⅔ cup sugar
- ½ cup fresh orange juice
- Grated zest of 1 orange
- 2 tablespoons hazelnut liqueur or 1½ teaspoons hazelnut extract
- ½ teaspoon orange extract
- 2 teaspoons pure vanilla extract
- 1½ teaspoons coffee extract
- Pinch of salt
- 1½ cups almond milk
- 1 teaspoon agar powder
- 1 tablespoon cornstarch

TOPPING:
- 3 tablespoons almond milk
- 2 tablespoons chocolate chips
- 1 teaspoon coffee extract
- ¼ cup roughly chopped, roasted hazelnuts

1. Drain the cashews and pour them into a blender along with the sugar, orange juice, orange zest, hazelnut liqueur, extracts, and

salt. Puree until very smooth and creamy. Make sure that no small bits of cashew remain; depending on how powerful your blender is, this could take 1 to 5 minutes.

2. In a medium-size saucepan, combine 1 cup of the almond milk and the agar powder. Bring to a rolling boil over high heat for 30 seconds, then reduce the heat to medium and simmer over for 5 minutes, stirring occasionally with a wire whisk.

3. Meanwhile, in a large measuring cup, whisk together the remaining ½ cup of almond milk with the cornstarch. Slowly pour it into the simmering almond milk mixture, stirring constantly for 3 to 4 minutes until thickened. Pour this hot mixture immediately into the cashew mixture in the blender and pulse until everything is smooth. Arrange the tart shells on a baking sheet and immediately pour equal amounts of hot filling into each shell. Let stand for 20 minutes; the agar will begin to set even at room temperature.

4. Once the filling has begun to set, prepare the topping. In a small saucepan over medium heat, bring the almond milk to a gentle simmer. Turn off the heat, sprinkle in the chocolate chips and coffee extract, and stir with a rubber spatula until the chips have melted and everything is smooth. Drizzle this chocolate mixture over the tarts: For neater drizzling, pour the topping into a clean squeeze bottle with a small-tip nozzle and carefully draw a zigzag pattern on top of each tart. You can also use a plastic bag with a tiny corner snipped out.

5. Sprinkle the tarts with a few chopped hazelnuts. Let them set at room temperature for another 5 minutes, then carefully move the tarts to the refrigerator to chill completely before serving.

❋ *Slices* ❋

Here's a make-ahead tip: Bake the tart shells up to 2 days before filling and store cooled shells in a tightly covered container on a kitchen counter until ready to use.

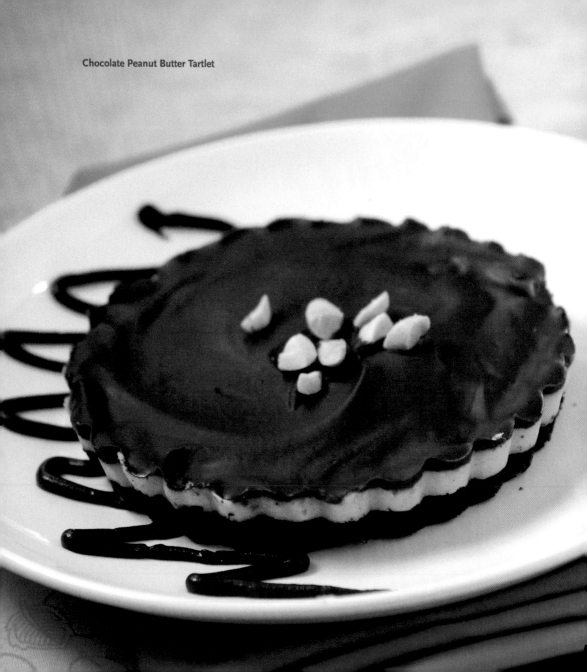

Chocolate Peanut Butter Tartlet

CHOCOLATE PEANUT BUTTER TARTLETS

MAKES SIX 4-INCH TARTS

AT LAST, A TART to please every chocolate and peanut butter lover in your life. To be fair, you may end up pleasing them too much and get repeated requests for these giant peanut butter cups, with a chocolate cookie crumb base and a fudgy chocolate topping—or spread the joy even more and make them *really* mini with our baby PB tart variation.

1 recipe GRAHAM CRACKER CRUST (page 46), Chocolate Cookie Crust variation

FILLING:
- 2 tablespoons nonhydrogenated margarine, lightly softened
- 2 tablespoons nonhydrogenated shortening
- ½ cup creamy, salted natural peanut butter
- 2 teaspoons pure vanilla extract
- 2 cups confectioner's sugar, sifted to remove any lumps
- 4 to 5 tablespoons almond milk

GANACHE:
- ⅓ cup almond milk
- 1 generous cup semisweet chocolate chips
- 2 tablespoons coconut oil

1. Preheat the oven to 350°F and lightly spray four 6-inch mini-tart pans with nonstick cooking spray. Distribute the crust mixture between the tart pans. Working from the edges first, firmly press the mixture into the bottom of the pan only (do not press it up along the sides). Place the tart pans on a baking sheet and bake for 10 minutes, then remove from the oven and let cool.

2. While the tarts are cooling, prepare the filling. In a large mixing bowl, use electric beaters to blend the margarine and the shortening until creamy, about 2 to 3 minutes. Beat in the peanut butter and the vanilla extract until smooth, then sift in the confectioner's sugar a little at a time until stiff but well blended. Now beat in the almond milk, one tablespoon at a time, until the filling is smooth and creamy like a thick frosting.

3. Dollop the filling into the cooled tart shells. Use a rubber spatula or lightly moistened fingertips to gently smooth the filling to the edges of the pan; take your time and make the tops as smooth as possible. Chill the tarts for half an hour.

4. Make the ganache: In a small saucepan, bring the almond milk to a rolling boil, then turn off the heat. Add the chocolate chips and coconut oil and use a rubber spatula to stir constantly until very smooth. Starting at the center of each chilled tart, spoon equal amounts of ganache on top, then smooth the ganache all the way to the edges.

5. Let the tarts cool for 10 minutes, then move them to the freezer and let chill for 6 hours or overnight. To remove a tart from its pan, do so when it's frozen and press the bottom from underneath and pop it free. Then, using the tip of a sharp knife, gently pry underneath the bottom of the crust to separate it from the pan. Let the tart stand at room temperature for 5 minutes before serving; for best results, serve tarts gently chilled.

Variation

CHOCOLATE PB MICROTARTS: If you have the time or inclination, you can make these into a dessert finger food! This makes around 96 tiny tarts, so it's an epic undertaking and needs to be reserved for special occasions, unless you have an afternoon to kill for absolutely no reason.

1. Preheat the oven to 350°F. Line mini-muffin tins with tiny liners. Squish a heaping teaspoon of crust into the liners and bake for 10 minutes. Remove from oven and let cool. Once cooled, remove from the tins and repeat with the remaining ingredients.

2. Add a heaping teaspoon of peanut butter filling to the crusts. Then spoon on a teaspoon of ganache and sprinkle with chopped peanuts. Let cool, and enjoy!

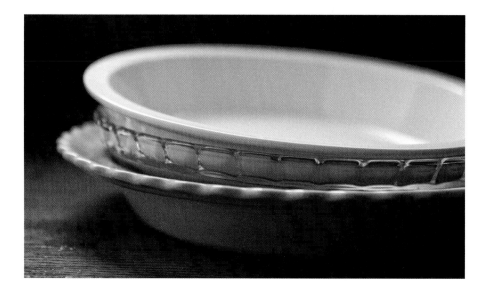

MANHATTAN MUD PIE

DO YOU ABSOLUTELY LOVE CHOCOLATE? This pie will make you prove it. It's rich and boozy and complete sloppy chocolate decadence, with a hint of coffee liqueur. The luscious pudding layer oozes all over the moist cake, so serve warm if you're looking for molten fudgy goodness (with a big scoop of vegan vanilla ice cream to melt in) or serve cold if you're craving a set pudding.

BOTTOM LAYER:

- 2 tablespoons cornstarch
- ¼ cup almond milk or your favorite nondairy milk
- 1 cup all-purpose flour
- ⅓ cup unsweetened cocoa powder
- ¾ teaspoon baking powder
- ¾ teaspoon salt
- ¾ cup sugar
- ½ cup coffee liqueur
- ⅓ cup canola oil
- 2 teaspoons pure vanilla extract

PUDDING LAYER:

- ⅓ cup cocoa powder
- ½ cup sugar
- 3 ounces bittersweet chocolate, finely chopped
- 1 cup boiling water
- ⅓ cup chocolate liqueur

1. Preheat the oven to 350°F. Start boiling the water for the pudding layer. Have ready a lightly greased 8-inch springform pan.

2. Prepare the bottom layer: In a mixing cup, vigorously stir the cornstarch into the almond milk until it's mostly dissolved. In a mixing bowl, sift together the flour, cocoa powder, baking powder, and salt. Mix in the sugar.

3. Make a well in the center of the dry ingredients and pour into it the cornstarch mixture, liqueur, oil, and vanilla extract. Mix until smooth. Spread the batter into the prepared pan and set aside.

4. Make the pudding layer: In a heatproof bowl, whisk together the cocoa powder, sugar, and chopped chocolate. Add the boiling water and mix with a fork until the chocolate has dissolved and the mixture is smooth. Mix in the liqueur and pour the pudding over the batter in the pan.

5. Bake the pie 45 to 50 minutes. Remove it from the oven and let cool just until the pan is at a temperature you can handle (the cake should still be hot). Move the cake to a serving plate and release the springform pan. Chocolate will ooze all over the cake. It's now ready to serve with a scoop of vegan vanilla ice cream.

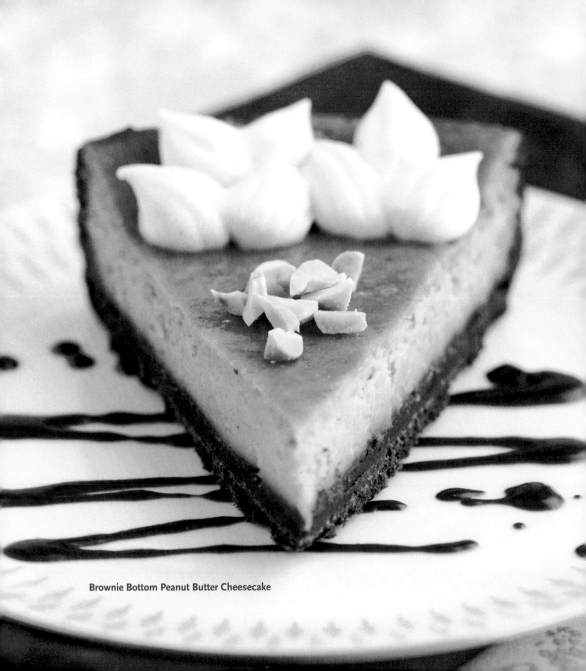

Brownie Bottom Peanut Butter Cheesecake

BROWNIE BOTTOM PEANUT BUTTER CHEESECAKE

MAKES ONE 9½-INCH CHEESECAKE

THIS IS IT, the ultimate dessert collision. Brownie. Peanut butter. Cheesecake! Never say we don't love you.

BROWNIE CRUST:

- 3 ounces semisweet chocolate
- 4 tablespoons nonhydrogenated margarine
- ½ cup sugar
- ¼ cup almond milk
- ½ teaspoon pure vanilla extract
- ⅔ cup all-purpose flour
- 3 tablespoons cocoa powder
- ½ teaspoon baking soda
- Pinch of salt

FILLING:

- ½ cup creamy salted natural peanut butter
- ⅓ cup ripe mashed banana (about 1 medium-size banana)
- 1 (12–14 ounce) package silken tofu, drained
- ⅔ cup sugar
- 2 tablespoons brown sugar
- 1 tablespoon coconut oil
- 4 teaspoons cornstarch
- 2 teaspoons lemon juice
- 2 teaspoons pure vanilla extract
- ¼ teaspoon salt

OPTIONAL GARNISH:

RAD WHIP (page 199) or store-bought vegan whipped topping and 3 tablespoons chocolate chips or chopped peanuts

1. Preheat the oven to 350°F. Generously spray the bottom and sides of a 9-inch springform pan with nonstick cooking spray. In a large microwave-safe bowl, heat the

chocolate for 1 minute. Stir and return it to the microwave for 30-second increments until completely melted, stirring after each 30 seconds. Be careful not to burn the chocolate. Add the margarine and stir with a rubber spatula until smooth.

2. Stir in the sugar, almond milk, and vanilla extract, then sift in the flour, cocoa powder, baking soda, and salt. Mix until smooth. Use the rubber spatula to spread the batter in an even layer into the bottom of the prepared pan. Bake for 8 minutes or until the top of the brownie looks puffed and crinkled, then move the pan to a cooling rack.

3. In a blender, puree all of the filling ingredients until very smooth. Pour the filling on top of the brownie crust. Carefully lift the pan about half an inch above a wooden cutting board and quickly bang it a few times to help release any large air bubbles from the batter.

4. Bake the cheesecake for 35 to 40 minutes until the top is lightly puffed and the edges of the cake are golden. Remove from the oven and let cool on a rack for 30 minutes. If garnishing with chocolate chips, press the chips in a decorative pattern on top of the hot cake. Move the cake to the fridge to complete cooling.

5. Don't even think about slicing this until the filling is absolutely cold, at least 4 hours or even better, overnight. Use a thin, sharp knife dipped in cold water to slice. Serve as is or garnish each slice with chopped peanuts, a dollop of Rad Whip, or chocolate shavings.

Variation

PEANUT BUTTER & JELLY CHEESECAKE: Omit the brownie crust and replace with GRAHAM CRACKER CRUST (page 46), prebake as directed. Top the peanut butter filling with ½ cup of melted strawberry jam, raspberry jam, or Concord grape jelly (see STRAWBERRY KIWI CRÈME TART, page 113, for melting instructions), dropping in random spoonfuls on top and using a chopstick to swirl a decorative pattern into the cake. If desired, decorate the cheesecake with a sprinkle of roughly chopped roasted peanuts. Bake and cool as directed.

☀ *Slices* ☀

◆ Making mini cheesecakes? Reduce the baking time for the crusts to 6 minutes and the total baking time to 25 to 30 minutes. The center of the cakes should jiggle slightly and not appear liquid.

◆ See page 94 for crack-free cheesecake baking!

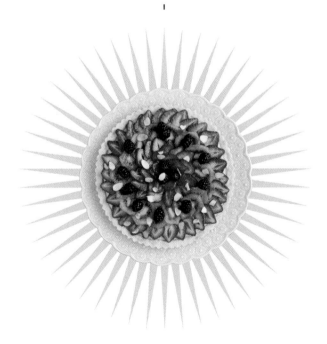

CAFÉ MOCHA CHEESECAKE

COFFEE AND CHOCOLATE need no introduction. But in case you need one, this cheesecake is a sublime grown-up treat for coffee breaks or really any break. Serve each slice with a dollop of RAD WHIP (page 199) or SWEET COCONUT CREAM (page 201) and garnish with a single chocolate-covered espresso bean.

1 recipe **GRAHAM CRACKER CRUST** (page 46) or Chocolate Cookie Crust or Black & White Crust variation

FILLING:
- ½ cup whole unroasted cashews, soaked in water for 2 to 8 hours or until very soft
- ½ cup well-mashed banana (about 2 medium-size bananas)
- 1 (12–14 ounce) package silken tofu, drained
- ¾ cup sugar
- 2 tablespoons coconut oil, room temperature
- 2 tablespoons instant espresso powder or instant coffee granules
- 2 teaspoons unsweetened cocoa powder

- 4 teaspoons cornstarch
- 1 tablespoon lemon juice
- 2 teaspoons pure vanilla extract
- ¼ teaspoon almond extract
- ¼ teaspoon salt
- ⅔ cup semisweet chocolate chips
- 1 tablespoon agave nectar

OPTIONAL GARNISH:
- RAD WHIP (page 199) and chocolate-covered espresso beans

1. Preheat the oven to 350°F. Lightly spray a 9-inch springform pan with cooking spray. Prepare the cookie crumb crust and press it very firmly into the pan. Bake for 10 minutes and move the pan to a

cooling rack. Leave the oven on, because you'll be baking the cheesecake in a bit.

2. Meanwhile, prepare the filling: Drain the cashews and blend with the banana, tofu, sugar, coconut oil, espresso powder, cocoa powder, cornstarch, lemon juice, vanilla and almond extracts, and salt. Blend the ingredients until completely smooth and no bits of cashew remain.

3. Set aside ⅔ cup of batter and pour the remaining batter onto the crust. Melt the chocolate chips over a double boiler or in a glass bowl in the microwave, stir with a spatula until smooth, and stir in the agave nectar. Pour the melted chocolate mixture into the reserved batter and stir very well until smooth. Spoon dollops of chocolate batter randomly on top of the cheesecake, then poke the end of a chopstick into a chocolate batter blob. Gently swirl the top to create a swirled pattern and

repeat with the remaining chocolate spots.

4. Bake the cheesecake for 45 to 50 minutes, until the top is lightly puffed and edges of cake are golden. Remove the cake from the oven and let it cool on a rack for 20 minutes, then move it to the fridge to complete cooling, at least 3 hours or even better, overnight. To serve, slice the cake with a thin, sharp knife dipped in cold water. Garnish each slice as desired and serve.

Variation

KAHLÚA & CREAM CHEESECAKE: At step 2, don't add the espresso powder just yet to the cheesecake batter. First, remove ⅔ cup of the batter from the blender and set aside, then add the espresso powder along with ¼ cup Kahlúa liqueur and the melted chocolate to the remaining batter in the blender, blend, and pour into the pan. Swirl the remaining white batter into the cheesecake as directed above.

GRASSHOPPER PIE

THE CLASSIC MINTY CHOCOLATE PIE, just as cute as you remember it. For best results use DeKuyper Crème de Menthe; it's vegan and a popular, easy-to-find brand of peppermint liqueur. The pie looks really adorable if you pipe whipped topping along the edge of the crust.

The mint flavor of this pie really blossoms after an overnight chilling in the fridge, and the coconut flavors mellow considerably, so try making this the night before your next chocolate mint pie soiree.

1 recipe **GRAHAM CRACKER CRUST** (page 46), Chocolate Cookie Crust variation, pressed into a greased 9-inch pie pan

FILLING:
- ½ cup whole unroasted cashews, soaked in water for 2 to 8 hours or until very soft
- 1 (13-ounce) can coconut milk, at room temperature
- ¼ cup crème de menthe
- ½ cup plain unsweetened almond milk
- ½ teaspoon agar powder
- ⅔ cup sugar
- ¼ cup coconut oil
- 2 teaspoons pure vanilla extract

- ½ teaspoon mint extract
- 1 to 2 drops green food coloring

DRIZZLE TOPPING:
- ¼ cup semisweet chocolate chips
- 2 teaspoons coconut oil

OPTIONAL GARNISH:
- **RAD WHIP** (page 199) or store-bought vegan whipped topping

1. Bake the crust for 10 minutes at 350°F, then remove from the oven and let cool.
2. Drain the cashews and place them

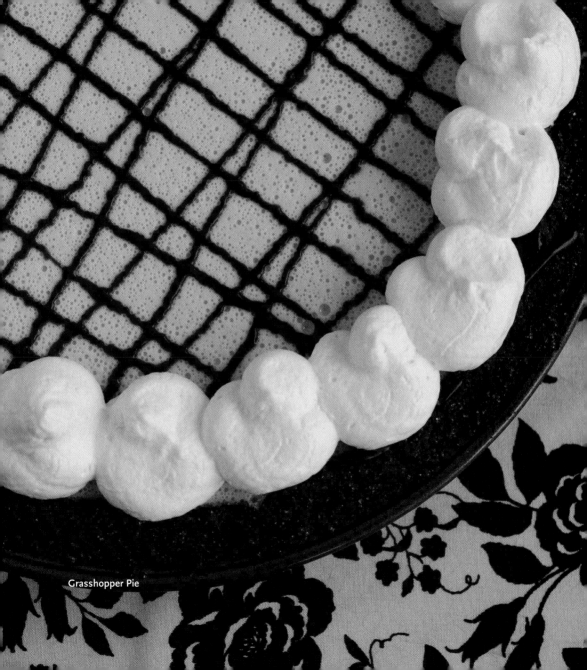
Grasshopper Pie

in a food processor or blender. Blend with the coconut milk and crème de menthe until totally smooth, scraping down the sides of the bowl occasionally. This can take up to 5 minutes depending on the strength of your machine.

3. In the meantime, stir together the almond milk and agar powder in a small (2-quart) saucepot. Bring the mixture to a boil, stirring consistently. Boil for 30 seconds, then lower the heat so that you're just getting small bubbles and cook for about 5 minutes, stirring occasionally. Whisk in the sugar. Add the coconut oil and mix until melted.

4. With the food processor running, stream the hot mixture in until thoroughly blended with the cashew mixture, then add the vanilla and mint extracts and food coloring. Pulse to combine.

5. Transfer the mixture to the prepared pie crust and refrigerate un-til set, about 4 to 6 hours. If there's a little extra filling, just put it in a cup to set and don't overfill the pie. The filling is very thin at first, but don't worry; that is how it's supposed to be!

6. When the pie is just about set, prepare the topping: In a bowl, microwave the chocolate chips using 50 percent power for 1½ to 2 minutes. Stir with a fork to thoroughly melt. Stir in the coconut oil to melt.

7. To assemble: With a rubber spatula, transfer the melted chocolate to a plastic bag. Snip the very corner of the bag (with as tiny a snip as you can manage) and drizzle the chocolate all over the pie in a zigzag or crisscross pattern.

8. Return the pie to the fridge to set for 20 minutes. If desired, pipe Rad Whip or vegan whipped topping around the edges of the pie, and serve!

CHOCOLATE MOUSSE TART

FEW CAN ARGUE with the power of perfectly rich (yet easy to prepare) vegan chocolate mousse; even fewer can resist it piled into a crisp chocolate tart shell. End a fancy dinner with slices atop plates garnished with fresh raspberries and a sprig of mint.

1 recipe **CHOCOLATE SHORTBREAD TART SHELL** (page 45) or **CHOCOLATE OLIVE OIL SHORTBREAD CRUST** (page 49), baked and cooled

FILLING:

- 1 (12–14 ounce) package silken tofu, drained
- ¼ cup plain soy milk
- 2 tablespoons pure maple syrup or agave nectar
- 1½ teaspoons pure vanilla extract
- 2 generous cups semisweet chocolate chips (one 12-ounce package)

GARNISH:

- Dark chocolate shavings or drizzle topping from **GRASSHOPPER PIE**, page 190 (see instructions below)
- Raspberries
- Fresh mint leaves

1. Crumble the tofu into a blender. Add the soy milk, maple syrup, and vanilla extract. Blend until very smooth. Melt the chocolate according to the directions on page 175, let it cool for 5 minutes. Add it to tofu mixture and pulse until creamy and smooth, stopping to scrape down the sides of the blender occasionally.

2. Pour the mixture into a large mixing bowl, cover with plastic wrap, and chill for 1 hour. The mousse should firm up but not be hard; if it's too stiff let it warm on the kitchen counter for 15 minutes.

3. To assemble the pie, use a rubber spatula to scoop the chocolate mousse into a very large pastry bag fitted with a large round nozzle with a ½-inch-wide opening or slightly bigger. Twist down the top of the bag to eliminate any air bubbles. Starting from the edge of the tart, pipe the mousse in a tight spiral until you reach the center. If you can't manage doing a huge spiral try piping big fat dots or use a big star tip and pipe fat stars. When the tart shell is filled, top with chocolate shavings

Slices

This tart looks adorable when piped into the tart shell, but if you don't happen to have the correct pastry tip for piping, you can pile it into the shell and then use a spatula to smooth it into a rounded mound, peaking in the middle.

or chill the tart for 30 minutes and then drizzle with chocolate drizzle topping. Garnish each individual slice with a few fresh raspberries and a sprig of mint.

4. Chill the tart for an hour before slicing with a thin, sharp knife dipped in cold water.

SALTED CHOCOLATE CARAMEL TART

MAKES 8 TO 10 SERVINGS

THIS SLIM TART packs maximum gooey coconut-caramel decadence into a buttery pastry shell, tasting kind of like an elegant Twix bar dusted with a whim of *fleur de sel* (or any fancy salt). A thin sliver per serving of this super-rich tart goes a long way.

1 recipe **SHORTBREAD TART SHELL** (page 44) or **CHOCOLATE SHORTBREAD TART SHELL** (page 45), fitted into a 10-inch tart pan and baked and cooled

COCONUT CARAMEL:
- 1½ cups sugar
- 3 tablespoons agave nectar
- ⅓ cup water
- ½ cup full-fat coconut milk
- 3 tablespoons nonhydrogenated margarine
- 1 teaspoon pure vanilla extract
- Pinch of salt

GANACHE:
- ⅓ cup coconut milk
- ¾ cup semisweet chocolate chips

- 1 tablespoon nonhydrogenated margarine

- About ⅛ teaspoon *fleur de sel* or other fancy, large-grained sea salt

Slices

This tart requires a little extra dessert-making skill; we recommend you hold off on trying this if you're new to baking or working with caramel. Also, this tart melts quickly in a warm environment. For best results and to avoid tragic tart melting, keep it chilled and let it warm only slightly for 5 minutes when ready to slice.

1. In a small (2-quart) saucepan with sides at least 4 inches high, add the sugar, agave nectar, and water. Don't stir the ingredients; instead hold the handle of the pan and gently swirl the pan a few times. Heat the mixture over high heat to bring it to a rolling, foaming boil. Cover and cook for 2 minutes, then lower the heat to medium. Continue to simmer until the mixture starts to turn a very pale golden color; this can take awhile, as long as 20 minutes, but when it starts, the caramel will begin to change color rapidly. Watch carefully as the mixture turns from light golden brown caramel color to a dark amber color and has thickened to almost soft ball stage (235°F on a candy thermometer). To test for soft ball, drizzle a drop of the caramel on a cold dish (place in the freezer for a few minutes to chill). When the caramel drop is completely cooled it should feel slightly firm but still yielding, like soft caramel candy. Stir in the coconut milk, margarine, vanilla extract, and salt; stand back as it will bubble and splatter just a little. Continue to stir and cook for 10 minutes, then turn off the heat.

2. Pour the caramel into the tart shell. Let stand for 10 minutes and then chill in the refrigerator for 30 minutes or until semifirm.

3. Prepare the ganache: In a small saucepan over medium heat, bring the coconut milk to a boil. Remove from heat and stir in the chocolate chips and margarine. Continue to stir until the chocolate has melted and the mixture is completely smooth and let stand for 5 minutes. Pour the ganache on top of the caramel and gently spread it to the edges; work quickly as the hot ganache may melt the caramel beneath.

4. Chill the tart for another 30 minutes, then sprinkle sparingly with *fleur de sel*. Continue to chill the tart until it's completely cold, at

least 4 hours or even better, overnight. To serve, remove the tart from the pan, then slice with a thin, sharp knife dipped in cold water. Keep the tart chilled until ready to serve.

Variation

BEER CARAMEL CHOCOLATE PRETZEL TART: Replace water with your favorite full-bodied, hoppy lager beer. Instead of sea salt, sprinkle with 2 tablespoons of crushed salted pretzels.

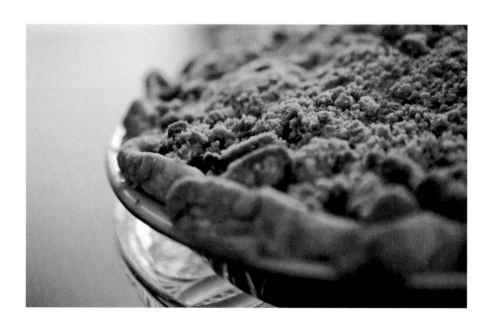

A FEW TOPPINGS

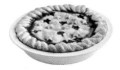

PIE NEEDS VERY FEW items to make it complete. Here are a few options for adding a creamy topping, or perhaps a drizzle of chocolate when the occasion calls for it.

RAD WHIP

SERVES 8

OMIGOD, VEGAN COOL WHIP! Yeah, there are a couple of good store-bought options these days, but this is really fun, makes a ton, and tastes incredibly fresh and creamy. It's better than cool; it's rad! Perfect for topping pies, puddings, ice cream sundaes, your finger, a spoon, and any place else whipped cream might be appropriate.

A few recipe notes: You blend this cream three times, once in the food processor or regular blender and then again with a hand mixer. Then it sets for a good long time and gets its final hand mixer whip. After it first sets in the freezer it looks a little rubbery and weird. Follow the directions and don't be alarmed! It will completely fluff up and smooth out when you blend it again, we promise; this is faerie unicorn tear magick here.

½ cup whole unroasted cashews, soaked in water for 2 to 8 hours or until very soft

⅓ cup coconut milk

1 cup plain unsweetened almond milk

¾ teaspoon agar powder

3 tablespoons sugar

2 tablespoons coconut oil plus 2 teaspoons

1 teaspoon pure vanilla extract

1. Place a large metal bowl in the freezer to chill; you'll be using it to blend up the Rad Whip so make sure it's big enough.

2. Drain the cashews and blend in a food processor or strong blender with the coconut milk and ½ cup of the almond milk until completely smooth. Rub the mixture between your fingers to make sure there is no graininess left; reaching this state could take up to 5 minutes depending on your machine.

3. In a small (2-quart) saucepan, heat the other ½ cup almond

milk, agar powder, and sugar. Bring to a boil and let simmer another 5 minutes, stirring occasionally. Add the coconut oil and stir to melt. It's important to make sure this doesn't set while on the stovetop, so be sure to have the blender mixture ready.

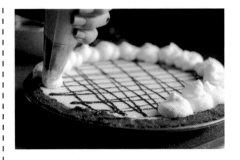

4. Stream the warm mixture into the blender or food processor with the machine turned on. Blend for about a minute on high to incorporate lots of bubbles, then add the vanilla extract and pulse to mix.

5. Transfer the mixture to the chilled metal bowl. Place in the freezer for about 30 minutes just to get it very very cold, but not frozen. When you remove it, it should be cold all the way through, and feel firm and even a bit rubbery. Don't worry! You did everything right . . . watch in amazement as it transforms.

6. Now take a hand mixer and beat like mad. The cream should start to soften and peaks should start to form, but it might take a minute or so. Once it is smooth and fluffy, cover it tightly with plastic wrap and place it back in the fridge to set again for at least 3 hours (the longer you let it set, the fluffier it will get, so if you let it set at least 8 hours or overnight, that is optimal). Now use a hand mixer one last time to get it even more fluffy.

7. Keep stored in a tightly sealed container for up to 5 days.

SWEET COCONUT CREAM

SERVES 8

THIS IS A SUPER-EASY way to get a thick, pourable cream, or a stiffer, scoopable cream if you have the patience to chill it for a few hours. Either way, it's a rich and decadent way to add creaminess to your fruit or chocolate pies.

1 can coconut milk (not lite)

½ cup confectioner's sugar

½ teaspoon pure vanilla extract

1. Refrigerate the can of coconut milk for at least 6 hours. When refrigerated, the cream from the coconut milk will rise to the top of the can and solidify. Open the can and scoop only the solid cream out into a mixing bowl, leaving the water behind. You can actually use that coconut cream as is, but we're going to whip and sweeten it for this.

2. Use a hand mixer to whip the cream, adding the confectioner's sugar bit by bit until completely incorporated. Once smooth and creamy, mix in the vanilla extract. Cover tightly with plastic wrap and refrigerate until ready to use. The longer it sits in the fridge, the stiffer it will get.

MACADAMIA CRÈME

MAKES 2 ½ CUPS

WE USE CASHEWS a lot in the book, but macadamias make a luscious cream as well. Because they're kind of pricey, we reserve them for special occasions and mix them with cashews. This cream is thick, but still pourable. It's especially fabulous with BASIL PEACH PIE (page 65)!

½ cup raw cashew pieces

½ cup roasted macadamias (if salted, rinse the salt off)

1½ cups almond milk or nondairy milk of your choice

1 teaspoon pure vanilla extract

1. Place the cashews and macadamias in a bowl and add enough water to cover them. Let the nuts soak for about 2 hours, and up to overnight, to soften. Drain well.

2. In a blender or food processor, grind up the nuts. Add the almond milk and vanilla extract and puree until smooth and not grainy. Depending on the strength of your device, it may take up to 5 minutes to get them very smooth, so be patient.

3. Place the mixture in a tightly sealed container and refrigerate for a few hours to set. The crème should be thick but pourable.

CHOCOLATE DRIZZLE

THIS IS THE EASIEST thing in the world, if you want to add some chocolate panache to your pie. Drizzle some sauce on vegan ice cream over fruit pie, or over whipped topping on an already chocolate pie. You can also spoon a little pool of chocolate onto the plate, and place the pie over it.

½ cup almond milk or nondairy milk of your choice

½ cup chocolate chips

1. In a small saucepan, bring the almond milk to a boil. Add the chocolate chips and lower the heat. Stir constantly with a rubber spatula until the chocolate is completely melted. Let the chocolate cool slightly before using.

METRIC CONVERSIONS

The recipes in this book have not been tested with metric measurements, so some variations might occur.

Remember that the weight of dry ingredients varies according to the volume or density factor: 1 cup of flour weighs far less than 1 cup of sugar, and 1 tablespoon doesn't necessarily hold 3 teaspoons.

GENERAL FORMULAS FOR METRIC CONVERSION

Ounces to grams	→	ounces x 28.35 = grams
Grams to ounces	→	grams x 0.035 = ounces
Pounds to grams	→	pounds x 453.5 = grams
Pounds to kilograms	→	pounds x 0.45 = kilograms
Cups to liters	→	cups x 0.24 = liters
Fahrenheit to Celsius	→	(°F − 32) x 5 ÷ 9 = °C
Celsius to Fahrenheit	→	(°C x 9) ÷ 5 + 32 = °F

VOLUME (LIQUID) MEASUREMENTS

1 teaspoon = ⅙ fluid ounce = 5 milliliters
1 tablespoon = ½ fluid ounce = 15 milliliters
2 tablespoons = 1 fluid ounce = 30 milliliters
¼ cup = 2 fluid ounces = 60 milliliters

⅓ cup = 2⅔ fluid ounces = 79 milliliters

½ cup = 4 fluid ounces = 118 milliliters

1 cup or ½ pint = 8 fluid ounces =
    250 milliliters

2 cups or 1 pint = 16 fluid ounces =
    500 milliliters

4 cups or 1 quart = 32 fluid ounces =
    1,000 milliliters

1 gallon = 4 liters

VOLUME (DRY) MEASUREMENTS

¼ teaspoon = 1 milliliter

½ teaspoon = 2 milliliters

¾ teaspoon = 4 milliliters

1 teaspoon = 5 milliliters

1 tablespoon = 15 milliliters

¼ cup = 59 milliliters

⅓ cup = 79 milliliters

½ cup = 118 milliliters

⅔ cup = 158 milliliters

¾ cup = 177 milliliters

1 cup = 225 milliliters

4 cups or 1 quart = 1 liter

½ gallon = 2 liters

1 gallon = 4 liters

WEIGHT (MASS) MEASUREMENTS

1 ounce = 30 grams

2 ounces = 55 grams

3 ounces = 85 grams

4 ounces = ¼ pound = 125 grams

8 ounces = ½ pound = 240 grams

12 ounces = ¾ pound = 375 grams

16 ounces = 1 pound = 454 grams

OVEN TEMPERATURE EQUIVALENTS, FAHRENHEIT (F) AND CELSIUS (C)

100°F = 38°C

200°F = 95°C

250°F = 120°C

300°F = 150°C

350°F = 180°C

400°F = 205°C

450°F = 230°C

LINEAR MEASUREMENTS

½ in = 1 ½ cm

1 inch = 2 ½ cm

6 inches = 15 cm

8 inches = 20 cm

10 inches = 25 cm

12 inches = 30 cm

20 inches = 50 cm

ACKNOWLEDGMENTS

Isa thanks John "Lazy Vegan" Mc-Devitt, as well as her family: Marlene Stewart, Michelle Moskowitz, Aaron Brown, Max & Norah.

Terry thanks John Stavropoulos for cleaning up the kitchen once more.

Terry and Isa would also like to thank: our publisher Katie McHugh, project manager Christine Marra, and agent Marc Gerald.

And we couldn't have done it without our Omaha pie team. Thank you to: Denise Muller for baking, ironing, and sweeping, Justin Limoges for photography, Gretchen Radler for the beautiful pies. Nor without Wednesday night's dedicated party of pie tasters: Dave Berg, Daniel Heacox, Todd Love, Jared Sorensen, and Matt Wilson, to name a few.

We always appreciate our testers, but with this book they really went above and beyond! Perfect creams, workshopping agar, and troubleshooting imperfect crusts, our testers worked day and night to make sure that each recipe was ready for your oven.

Thank you guys, we really love you!

Kristen Blackmore
Michelle Cavigliano
Mel Chang

Erin Goddard
Cara Heberling
Teressa Jackson
Mo Martin

Megan McClellan
Allison Nordahl
Thalia Palmer
Dayna Rozental

Jess Scone
Sarah Willson
Elizabeth Wood

ACKNOWLEDGMENTS

Not Shown:

Keren Form

Amy Gedgaudas

Gabrielle Pope

Stephanie Roy

Amanda Sacco

Katie Schultz

Claudia Weber

Danielle Leda White

Kirstin Wilson

INDEX

A

Agar flakes, 8–9

Agar powder (agar-agar), 7–9

Almonds, Press-In Almond Crust/
variation, 52

Apple cider vinegar
gluten and, 13, 26
making crusts and, 13, 26

Apples
Apple Brown Betty/variation, 130–131
Apple Cream Raisin Pie, 128–129
Apple Crisp, 135–136
Appleberry Pie/variation, 70–72
Cosmos Apple Pie, 125–127
Figgy Apple Hand Pies, 137–138
French Toast Apple Cobbler, 132–134

Arrowroot, 7

B

Bananas
Banana Cookie Cream Pudding/
variation, 122–123

Banana Kahlúa Cheesecake
(variation recipe), 94

Banana Split Cheesecake (variation
recipe), 94

Banana Toffee Pudding Pie (Banoffee
Pie)/variation, 114–116

Chocolate Galaxy Banana
Cheesecake/variations, 92–94

Banoffee pie
about, 114
Banana Toffee Pudding Pie (Banoffee
Pie)/variation, 114–116
Coffee Banoffee Pie, 116

Basil
Basil Peach Pie, 64–66
tips, 66

Beer Caramel Chocolate Pretzel Tart,
197

Beet sugar, 9

Berries
Appleberry Pie/variation, 70–72
Pearberry Pie (variation recipe), 72

ABOUT THE AUTHORS

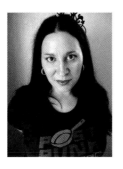 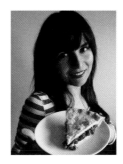

ISA CHANDRA MOSKOWITZ & TERRY HOPE ROMERO

are award-winning vegan chefs and authors of several best-selling cookbooks, including *Veganomicon* and *Vegan Cupcakes Take Over the World*. They host the Web site *The Post Punk Kitchen* at www.theppk.com.